One Hundred Years
of Heroin

One Hundred Years of Heroin

EDITED BY DAVID F. MUSTO

*With the assistance of Pamela Korsmeyer
and Thomas W. Maulucci, Jr.*

AUBURN HOUSE
Westport, Connecticut • London

Library of Congress Cataloging-in-Publication Data

One hundred years of heroin / edited by David F. Musto with the assistance of Pamela Korsmeyer and Thomas W. Maulucci, Jr.
  p. cm.
  Includes bibliographical references and index.
  ISBN 0–86569–309–9 (alk. paper)—ISBN 0–86569–324–2 (pbk. : alk. paper)
  1. Heroin habit—United States—History. 2. Heroin habit—Treatment—United States—History. I. Musto, David F., 1936– II. Korsmeyer, Pamela, 1945– III. Maulucci, Thomas W.
HV5825.O63 2002
363.29′3—dc21   2001053836

British Library Cataloguing in Publication Data is available.

Library of Congress Catalog Card Number: 2001053836
ISBN: 0–86569–309–9
    0–86569–324–2 (pbk.)

First published in 2002

Auburn House, 88 Post Road West, Westport, CT 06881
An imprint of Greenwood Publishing Group, Inc.
www.greenwood.com

Printed in the United States of America

The paper used in this book complies with the
Permanent Paper Standard issued by the National
Information Standards Organization (Z39.48–1984).

10 9 8 7 6 5 4 3 2 1

The chapter by Peter Reuter and Robert MacCoun was published, in slightly altered form, in
Drug War Heresies: Learning from Other Vices, Times, and Places by Robert J. MacCoun and
Peter Reuter, copyright © 2001 by Robert J. MacCoun and Peter Reuter (New York:
Cambridge University Press, 2001).

This book is dedicated to the memory of
Robert S. Byck, M.D. (1933–1999)

Contents

Preface

Heroin, one of the most feared and yet desired drugs in the world, is not a natural product but, rather, an achievement of organic chemistry. In the first decade of the nineteenth century morphine was isolated from crude opium, and in the 1870s an acetylized compound was synthesized from morphine. In the last decade of that century the Bayer Pharmaceutical Company studied the new compound intensively, and in 1898 presented it to the world, under the brand name *heroin*, as a cough suppressant. Since then, heroin has been used globally for its mind-altering effects; its powers as a cough suppressant are now reflected only in the manner in which death from overdose occurs: respiratory depression. Over the past century millions of persons have become addicted to heroin. Through manufacturing and distributing this product, criminal cartels in some parts of the world have acquired so much money and power that they have been able to destabilize governments.

This book is an attempt to understand the evolution of heroin from its introduction as a useful and important medicine to its role as a drug whose image everywhere conjures either disgust or desire. The chapters arise from a conference held in New Haven on September 19, 1998—precisely one hundred years after the commercial introduction of heroin. That gathering brought together a remarkable set of experts on heroin's history and effects, and on related social policies.

Acknowledgments

This book grew out of a conference at Yale that marked the centennial of heroin's introduction to medical practice. Through extensive planning and precise execution, my research associates Pamela Korsmeyer and Thomas Maulucci smoothly organized the meeting. Keith Lostaglio, then a graduate student in the history of medicine, skillfully negotiated arrangements for the venue. I am most grateful to the speakers, in particular to Senator Daniel Patrick Moynihan, who opened the conference.

Ms. Korsmeyer and Mr. Maulucci later began to shepherd the transformation of talks into chapters. The project was then assumed by Cynthia Wells, who had extensive experience at the Yale University Press. She joined our group as a research associate and carefully edited the text for publication. Gretchen Kreuger, a graduate student in the history of medicine, assisted Ms. Wells with energy, precision, and resourcefulness. At Greenwood Press, Jane Garry has been, from the start, encouraging and invariably helpful.

This book is dedicated to Robert Byck, M.D., Professor of Psychiatry and Pharmacology at Yale Medical School and a friend for two decades. Bob's interests included the history of cocaine, a substance he also had studied clinically. A telling example of his insight into drugs and society was his warning to Congress in 1979 that America was on the verge of a crisis in cocaine smoking, which indeed came to pass and later was called the crack epidemic. I hope that the thoughts and findings gathered here will assist other such dedicated scholars, clinicians, and policy makers.

The editor gratefully acknowledges the research support made possible through grant number K05DA00219-08 from the National Institute on Drug Abuse.

Introduction:
The Origins of Heroin

David F. Musto

Heroin is a trade name coined by the Bayer Pharmaceutical Company when diacetylmorphine was marketed in 1898. The story of this product begins in 1803, when F. W. A. Sertürner, a pharmacist in Paderborn, Germany, isolated a new narcotic substance from the juice of the opium poppy. Named after Morpheus, the god of sleep, morphine was being produced in various locations, including Philadelphia, by the 1830s, and by midcentury had become a mainstay for controlling pain. As the century progressed, chemists experimented with the morphine molecule, in hopes of improving the drug. They were concerned not only about the emergence of such side effects as nausea, vomiting, and constipation but also about the increasingly apparent possibility of addiction. A second area of interest was one of morphine's positive attributes, its ability—similar to that of another ingredient of crude opium, codeine—to weaken the cough reflex. At the time, pneumonia and tuberculosis were leading causes of illness and death, and there was a great need for a more effective cough suppressant. Although such an analgesic would not cure these serious pulmonary ailments, it would allow rest from persistent, unproductive coughing, which would comfort the sufferer and aid in healing.

The earliest known synthesis of diacetylmorphine occurred in 1874 when Charles Alder White at St. Mary's Hospital Medical School in London created a number of esters of morphine. (The account that follows in the next several paragraphs relies largely on Sneader 1998.) Experiments on animals, however, were not particularly significant. Then, in 1888 at Edinburgh, David Dott and Ralph Stockman reported that diacetylmorphine was stronger than morphine. Further studies in 1890 on frogs and rabbits indicated that the new compound was more powerful than morphine in depressing the respiratory center but had a lower narcotic (or sleep-inducing) effect. No clinical application seems to have followed these pharmacological papers.

In 1898 Joseph von Mering reported on a series of morphine derivatives for the Merck Pharmaceutical Company, which had been among those searching for a cough suppressant. As a result of von Mering's research, Merck had fixed upon ethylmorphine and had begun to market it in January 1898 under the name *dionin*. Dionin was the first derivative of morphine to enter the commercial market. Von Mering had dismissed diacetylmorphine, maintaining that it could not equal morphine's ability to suppress coughing nor to relieve pain.

Meanwhile, researchers at Bayer had discovered that some drugs could be made more palatable by adding an acetyl group to the original molecule. For example, Bayer had developed and marketed *tannigen*, which added two acetyl groups to tannic acid, as an antidiarrheal. Salicylic acid, used for joint pain, was irritating to the stomach. Bayer chemists added to it an acetyl group, resulting in a new and remarkable product, which the company named *aspirin*.

On August 21, 1897, two weeks after he had synthesized sodium acetylsalicylic acid, later marketed as *aspirin*, Felix Hoffmann, a researcher at the Bayer laboratory, synthesized diacetylmorphine, making possible further studies of that morphine derivative. Walter Sneader of the University of Strathclyde has pointed out that Hoffmann's synthesis of diacetylmorphine occurred before the publication of von Mering's paper and four months before the introduction of dionin. Therefore, it appears to have been an original investigation, not one undertaken in competition with Merck. Nor could Hoffmann have seen and possibly have been discouraged by von Mering's negative description of diacetylmorphine.

At about this time Heinrich Dreser was appointed head of Bayer's pharmacological laboratories. Dreser soon began experimenting on animals, using Hoffmann's morphine derivative as a substitute for codeine to suppress the cough reflex. He reported his results to the Congress of German Natural Scientists and Physicians on September 19, 1898, a date that could be considered the "birthday" of heroin. Omitting any reference to the work of earlier investigators, Dreser announced his own impressive clinical results, which indicated that the compound not only reduced the cough reflex but also appeared to strengthen respiration. Although breathing slowed, it became deeper and more effective. It was as if diacetylmorphine had a specific effect on the lungs similar to that of digitalis on the heart. As Gregory Higby has pointed out, many physicians confirmed this positive effect on the lungs in the years immediately following heroin's introduction (Higby 1986, 138). Belief that heroin could aid respiration seemed to underlie Bayer's enthusiasm for the drug, although a decade or so later the stimulant effect would be shown to be a misperception.

In June 1898 Bayer registered the name *heroin* for its preparation of diacetylmorphine. The origin of this trade name is debated, but a reasonable explanation is that it is derived from the German word *heroisch*, which, when applied to a medicine, means "strong." Indeed, heroin is about twice as strong as morphine by weight.

During 1898 the Bayer laboratory published at least three papers on heroin, one of which is described by Sneader as "the most extensive scientific paper yet to have emerged from any industrial pharmacological laboratory" (Sneader 1998, 1698). Medical periodicals soon included many papers on heroin, almost all of which were laudatory (see Higby 1986, 138). Theobald Floret, the Bayer Company physician, reported favorably on the use of heroin in sixty cases, including instances of pharyngitis, tracheitis, bronchitis, and pulmonary tuberculosis. He gave heroin in powder or pill form in doses ranging from 5 to 10 mgm, three to four times a day, not to exceed 10 mgm in a single dose or 20 mgm in a day (Floret 1899).

Considering the current image of heroin, we should note that the issue of addiction was not overlooked. In 1899 Floret assured the medical profession in these words: "I have treated many patients for weeks with heroin, without one observation that it may lead to dependency; in these cases, equal doses in the beginning and end had the same effect" (Floret 1899, 6). Georg Strube, however, writing in the *Berliner klinische Wochenschrift* in 1898, had doubts. He feared that morphinism, the contemporary term for the addiction, might be followed by heroinism. He argued that heroin should be used "only under medical control, and not dispensed too generously, so that, despite its good effect when used for proper indications, it does not fall into discredit through misuse or indolence" (8). Yet numerous reports found almost no problem with heroin and praised it for lacking morphine's undesirable side effects while providing almost uniformly successful results. For example, A. Holtkamp, writing in the *Deutschen medizinischen Wochenschrift* in 1898, asserted that he had not had a single unfavorable result in 187 cases ranging from hip pain to insomnia, and concluded that "heroin [is] an extraordinary remedy which far surpasses morphine in speed and certainty of effect and, above all, by the lack of bad side effects and consequences" (14). A few physicians told of using heroin to wean morphine addicts from that opiate, and some in later generations would mistakenly believe that this had been the reason for heroin's introduction.

Warnings about heroin's own addictive properties, however, started to accumulate. Interestingly, one of the earliest came from an American authority writing in the first volume of *Merck's Archive*. Professor H. C. Wood of the University of Pennsylvania warned of possible addictiveness in 1899. His caution was echoed the following year in the *American Yearbook of Medicine and Surgery*, which acknowledged heroin's value as a cough suppressant but warned that "for the present, small doses should be used and administered with some care, as the toxic properties of the drug are not thoroughly well known." In 1906 the American Medical Association severely warned the profession that "the [heroin] habit is readily formed and leads to the most deplorable results" (Musto, 1974, 176).

By 1912 heroin-related admissions to Philadelphia and New York hospitals were rising rapidly. Among recreational drug users, heroin had become popular as a replacement for morphine. At Bellevue Hospital in New York, heroin surpassed morphine as the primary cause of addiction admissions by 1915 (Musto 1974, 178-79).

From the time of the surge in admissions, heroin's path moved swiftly toward prohibition. By 1919 heroin had become so popular among teenage male gangs in New York City that the health commissioner coined the phrase "the American disease" to describe the phenomenon. In 1921 a federal statute banned importation of manufactured narcotics (morphine, cocaine, heroin, and so forth) and permitted the importation of only crude opium and coca leaves, from which American manufacturers would make the drugs.

As a result of growing fear of heroin, in 1924 manufacture of the drug from crude opium was prohibited, although it remained at least theoretically possible for a physician to prescribe heroin and, if there was a pharmacist who still had a supply, to have it dispensed. This provision was eliminated by the Narcotic Control Act of 1956, which required that anyone who had a supply of heroin turn it over to the government within three months. Subsequently heroin stocks would be considered contraband. For many years, the only legal way to obtain heroin has been to be granted a license for experimentation from the Food and Drug Administration.

In the following chapters, the contributors to this volume will take up the story of heroin in America: its medical history and cultural image; its place in health policy and criminal law; its appearance, diminishment, and reemergence as a social problem over the course of a century.

ACKNOWLEDGMENT

The author gratefully acknowledges the help of Cassandra Kniffin and Peter and Annette Wegener in translating essays from the German.

REFERENCES

Floret, Theobald. 1899. "Weiteres über Heroin." *Therapeutische Monatshefte* no. 6 (June).

Higby, Gregory J. 1986. "Heroin and Medical Reasoning: The Power of Analogy." *New York State Journal of Medicine* 86, no. 3 (March): 137–42.

Holtkamp, A. 1899. "Weitere Mittheilungen über therapeutische Versuche mit Heroin." *Deutschen medizinischen Wochenschrift* no. 14.

Kniffin, Cassandra L. 1990. "The Story of Heroin: The Power of Perception." Unpublished paper.

Musto, David F. 1974. "Early History of Heroin in the United States." In *Addiction*. Edited by Peter G. Bourne. New York: Academic Press.

Sneader, Walter. 1998. "The Discovery of Heroin." *Lancet* 352: 1697–99.

Strube, Georg. 1898. "Mittheilung über therapeutische Versuche mit Heroin." *Berliner klinische Wochenschrift* no. 45.

Part I

The First Sixty Years

The Roads to H:
The Emergence of the American
Heroin Complex, 1898–1956

David T. Courtwright

For some years I have been working on a history of the reception and impact of novel psychoactive drugs. The other day it occurred to me that, at bottom, the story is really a very simple one. It is that of the sorcerer's apprentice. Promising new drugs—aqua vitae, tobacco, morphine, cocaine, barbiturates, amphetamines—are introduced. Therapeutic claims are made and evaluated. Doctors argue among themselves about indications, dosage, and toxicity. The intramural debates seldom attract public notice. But, sooner or later, the new drug slips the bonds of medical discourse and control. It escapes into a larger world of popular pleasure and mischief, prompting official intervention.

The history of heroin in the United States fits neatly into this pattern. In 1898 it was just another promising new product from the Bayer Pharmaceutical Company. In the 1910s it developed a growing underworld following and by the 1920s had become the mainstay of the black market. The federal government outlawed the manufacture of heroin in 1924; as existing stocks dwindled to a few hundred ounces, the drug virtually disappeared from medical practice. The last remaining supplies were swept up by the Narcotic Control Act of 1956, which required the surrender of all remaining pharmaceutical heroin to the federal government. Heroin became, so to speak, America's first Schedule I drug. Its use was totally prohibited except for restricted research purposes, as cannabis, LSD-25, DMT, and mescaline would be in later years. However, the fact that heroin shared the fate of other potent psychoactive drugs is not an adequate explanation of its prohibition. We need to look more closely at the process of its transformation. We need to understand precisely when, how, and why heroin became H, the top enforcement priority of the Bureau of Narcotics and the basis of an underworld subculture—predominantly white before World War II, and minority thereafter.

MEDICAL USE AND ADDICTION

Heroin use and addiction were originally medical phenomena. What is not generally understood, however, is that the percentage of medical addicts who used heroin was never large. A retrospective study of fifty mostly medical cases published in 1918 showed only two heroin users, or 4 percent of the total (Scheffel 1918, 853–54). Lawrence Kolb, the government's leading medical authority on addiction, carried out a similar study of 150 medical addicts whose use began between 1898 and 1924, that is, after heroin was introduced and before it was effectively outlawed in the United States. The result: two heroin cases, or just 1.3 percent of the total. "My idea has been that the use of heroin in medical practice seldom resulted in addiction," Kolb wrote, "although when used in the underworld for dissipation only it doubtless has produced numerous addicts."[1]

The infrequency of iatrogenic heroin addiction was due to several factors. Heroin, in contrast to morphine and cocaine, was not touted for virtually every physical and medical affliction. Heroin was discussed in the medical literature primarily as a cough suppressant and means of alleviating respiratory distress. It was "recommended chiefly for the treatment of the air passages attended with cough, difficult breathing and spasm, such as different forms of bronchitis, pneumonia, consumption, asthma, whooping cough, laryngitis, and certain forms of hay fever," summed up a 1906 JAMA literature review ("Heroin Hydrochloride" 1906, 1303). While some authorities also recommended the drug as an analgesic, this idea was controversial, and early on was challenged by several German and American authorities (for example, Floret 1896, 512; Manges 1898, 770; and Wood 1899, 89–90).[2]

Advertising stressed heroin as a specific for respiratory symptoms. This was true even when heroin was combined with other analgesic products such as Antikamnia, a popular medication whose name means "against pain." The promotional literature for Antikamnia and heroin mentioned several possible indications, but concentrated on glowing clinical reports of cases involving cough and respiratory ailments. The medication came in the form of a tablet consisting of 5 grains of Antikamnia (47 parts acetanilid, 50 parts sodium bicarbonate, and 3 parts tartaric acid) and just 1/12 grain (5 mg) of heroin.[3]

This was typical. When heroin was prescribed for cough and respiratory ailments, it was given in small doses in tablets, pills, pastilles, elixirs, or glycerin solutions. Some preparations contained only 1 or 2 mg per dose (see, e.g., "Herotopine" and "Hermonal," n.d., W. H. Schieffelin and Company Collection). The ingestion of small amounts of an opiate was a good deal safer, from the standpoint of addiction, than hypodermic injection, which was how morphine was often administered.

Death was also a good protection against addiction. Pneumonia and tuberculosis had particularly high mortality rates in the period before antibiotics. Patients with these conditions who were treated with heroin presumably would not have lasted long as addicts, assuming they reached the point of physical dependence.

While some early reports gave assurances that heroin was not habit-forming, and even recommended it as a treatment for morphine addiction, physicians were quickly disabused of these notions. By early 1900 there were several cautionary statements about heroin's toxic and habit-forming potential; by 1903, if not sooner, there were firm and unambiguous declarations with such titles as "The Heroin Habit: Another Curse" (Pettey 1903; see also Wood 1899, 90; Manges 1900, 82; and "Caution Regarding Heroin" 1900, 44).

These warnings about iatrogenic heroin addiction came sooner than comparable warnings about morphine. They were received by physicians who were better educated, more therapeutically conservative, and more mindful of specific treatments for specific diseases than their counterparts of the 1870s and 1880s, when morphine reigned as panacea. In fact, most American (and, ironically, German) doctors in private practice eventually became so wary of heroin that they gave up prescribing it before they were legally required to do so. Government and military physicians had less choice in the matter. The U.S. Public Health Service ceased dispensing heroin in 1916; the army, in 1923; the navy, in 1924 (see "Symposium on 'The Doctor and the Drug Addict'" 1920, 1591; New York State Narcotic Drug Control Commission 1920, 41; Wolff 1932, 2180; and Anslinger 1936).

Now contrast the heroin situation with that of aspirin. Introduced commercially in 1899, the year after heroin, aspirin was Bayer's best-selling drug by 1906 and one of the most widely prescribed drugs in the world by 1914 (McTavish 1987, 104).[4] Not only was aspirin useful in treating a wide variety of conditions, but it was relatively safe and not habit-forming (in the sense of physical dependence). Indeed, I have long believed that one of the reasons for the decline of all forms of iatrogenic opiate addiction in the early twentieth century was the availability of aspirin and kindred preparations to treat rheumatism, colds and flu, toothaches and headaches, and other common aches and pains.

Going further, I believe that degree of exposure is the single most crucial variable in accounting for the prevalence of heroin or any other type of addiction. Yes, set and setting matter; and yes, personality and genetic makeup play a role; and yes, social integration and cultural norms can militate against abuse; and yes, only a minority of those exposed to a given drug typically end up as full-blown addicts. The simple fact remains, however, that those who are never exposed to a drug will never become addicted, and those who are seldom exposed are at much lower risk than those frequently exposed. Aspirin reduced the odds that millions of people from all walks of life who were suffering from common afflictions would come into contact, through either prescription or self-medication, with powerful opiates like morphine or heroin. The net effect was less opiate addiction.

NONMEDICAL USE AND ADDICTION

How, then, were nonmedical users exposed? No simple answer is possible here. In the underworld, many roads led to H. One story has it that prisoners in a state penitentiary were given heroin for cough. News spread among the inmates that the cough pills were "good dope." Word spread outside the prison, and eventually to tenderloins all over the country (Kane et al. 1917, 503).[5] The story is plausible except in one detail. It seems more likely that word of heroin's psychoactive potency spread from multiple sites, rather than one particular prison.

We know that nonmedical heroin addiction was definitely in play by 1910, the year when Leroy Street, pseudonymous author of *I Was a Drug Addict*, and his teenage friends first started sniffing the drug (Street 1953, 11).[6] We also know that many of the early nonmedical heroin users—mostly sniffers—had previously used other drugs, notably opium, cocaine, and tobacco cigarettes.

Police pressure and a national import ban (enacted 1909) had made opium smoking riskier and more expensive. Heroin sniffing was cheaper, quicker, and much harder to detect. By 1916 several reports described opium smokers who had expediently switched to heroin (see, e.g., Bailey 1916, 314; and McIver and Price 1916, 477, 478). Something similar happened with cocaine. The illicit market for cocaine existed well before passage of the 1914 Harrison Narcotic Act. It was created by a combination of informal professional controls—druggists wouldn't sell cocaine to just anybody—and proliferating legal controls of varying stringency (Spillane 2000). The result was an illicit market and higher prices. Decks of cocaine retailed on the streets of New York City for 25 cents, but contained only 1.3 grains (< 85 mg), making the actual price eleven times that of the legitimate wholesale price (Musto 1990, 322–23).

Heroin, by contrast, was cheaper and more readily available from druggists. "Dope users have turned to [heroin]," Boston reformers complained in 1912, "and as the drug is not so well known we find apothecaries who would not sell cocaine who are selling heroin apparently quite freely" (Chase et al. 1912, 9; see also Towns 1916, 221). Heroin was taken in the accustomed form, sniffing; didn't require injection; and had the added advantage of alleviating unpleasant symptoms, such as depression, that might be experienced when quitting cocaine. In 1923 Lawrence Kolb began a systematic study of 230 cases of narcotic addiction, including 40 heroin addicts. His records show that twenty-six of the forty heroin cases used cocaine prior to or concurrently with their first use of heroin (Kolb Papers, Box 6; Courtwright 1982, 161–62 n. 9; see also Stokes 1918, 756–57; Farr 1915, 893–94).

Not all of the heroin sniffers were veteran opium or cocaine users. Another type was the teenage working-class boy, often of immigrant parents, who lived in a "dirty, noisy, cheap, and tough" neighborhood (Stokes 1918, 757). He began using heroin out of curiosity or peer pressure after he had been introduced by someone in his "gang"—more like a younger, scruffier version of the Bowery Boys than the Crips or the Bloods. If he took any other drug on a regular basis, it was tobacco. No observation about the first generation of nonmedical heroin addicts is more commonplace than that they were inveterate cigarette smokers (e.g., Blanchard 1913, 142; and Stokes 1918: 756).

Is there a connection? The chronology, geography, and sociology are all suggestive. Cigarette use was exploding at the same time nonmedical heroin use was taking off. New York City, the center of heroin use, was also the center of the cigarette revolution. In 1910 the city accounted for 25 percent of all U.S. cigarette sales, despite having only about 5 percent of the U.S. population. Cigarettes were particularly popular with New York's immigrants—and many heroin addicts, though born in the United States, came from immigrant families.[7]

Theories developed. R. M. Blanchard, an army doctor, speculated that inhaling smoke increased the absorption of heroin (Blanchard 1913, 142). Harvey Wiley argued that the boy who acquired the cigarette habit would be "brought into sympathetic association with boys who are going to the bad" and that, among other things, he would "more readily become a victim of alcohol, cocain [sic], opium, and other narcotic drugs"—an early version of the gateway theory.[8] The addiction specialist Charles Towns likewise argued that cigarettes to alcohol to opiates was a natural progression, both because smokers developed a need for stimulation and because they ran with bad companions (Towns 1916, 152–53, 167, 172).[9] It is hard to know how much weight to assign cigarettes in the etiology equation, but it is at least plausible that their growing use—even more a symbol of defiance and deviance in 1910 than today—by groups of teenage boys paved the way for heroin experimentation.

HEROIN OUTLAWED

The emerging stereotype of the heroin addict was far more frightening than that of the old-fashioned morphine addict. Heroin addicts were boys and young men who ruined themselves in the prime of life. Morphine addicts were older and sicker and more often female. Heroin addiction was a vice. Morphine addiction had often originated in response to pain or chronic disease. Heroin addicts were dumb, greedy for drugs, visible, and rude, "members of gangs who congregate on street corners particularly at night, and make insulting remarks to people who pass." Morphine addicts were "more intelligent, secretive as to their habit, and usually temperate in the dosage of their drug" (Leahy 1915, 256; Stokes 1918, 757). Heroin addicts came from the lower and "criminal" classes of the big cities. Morphine addicts came from more diverse and, on the whole, better social backgrounds. The data in figure 1.1, based on Treasury Department questionnaires, show where nearly ten thousand addicts were institutionalized during the period 1916–1918 (U.S. Treasury Department 1919, 15–19). Heroin addicts were more numerous than morphine addicts in jails and prisons, while morphine addicts were far more numerous than heroin addicts in private hospitals and sanatoria. Unsurprisingly, opium smokers and cocaine addicts were also concentrated in penal or public institutions.

Subsequent studies showed a similar pattern. Of 632 convicted male addicts judged suitable for custodial treatment at New York City's Correction Hospital from March 1927 to June 1928, 588 (93 percent) used heroin alone or in combination with other drugs. Of 200 female addicts, 168 (84 percent) did likewise. Though straight morphine addicts were still common in the South in the late 1920s, they were increasingly rare in the North, particularly in correctional settings (Tuttle n.d.).

Why were so many heroin addicts behind bars? In objective terms, the answers are plain enough: because they stole or dealt drugs to support their habits; because they were reared in the slums; because they were single males in their teens and twenties, "prime time" for crime with or without drugs. But inventive propagandists like Richmond P. Hobson gave another answer: because of the action of heroin itself. It "exalted the ego," he testified, making the addict "suited for daring crimes, holdups, robberies, and such crimes as bandits of old never dared" (U.S. Senate, Committee on Printing 1924, 17).[10] Even if heroin addicts did not commit crimes, they were dangerous because of their tendency to proselytize (Bailey 1916, 315). "He has a mania to see others become addicts," said Hobson, who quoted with approval a

Figure 1.1
Institutionalized Addicts, 1916–1918 (9,822 Cases available to Treasury Dept.)

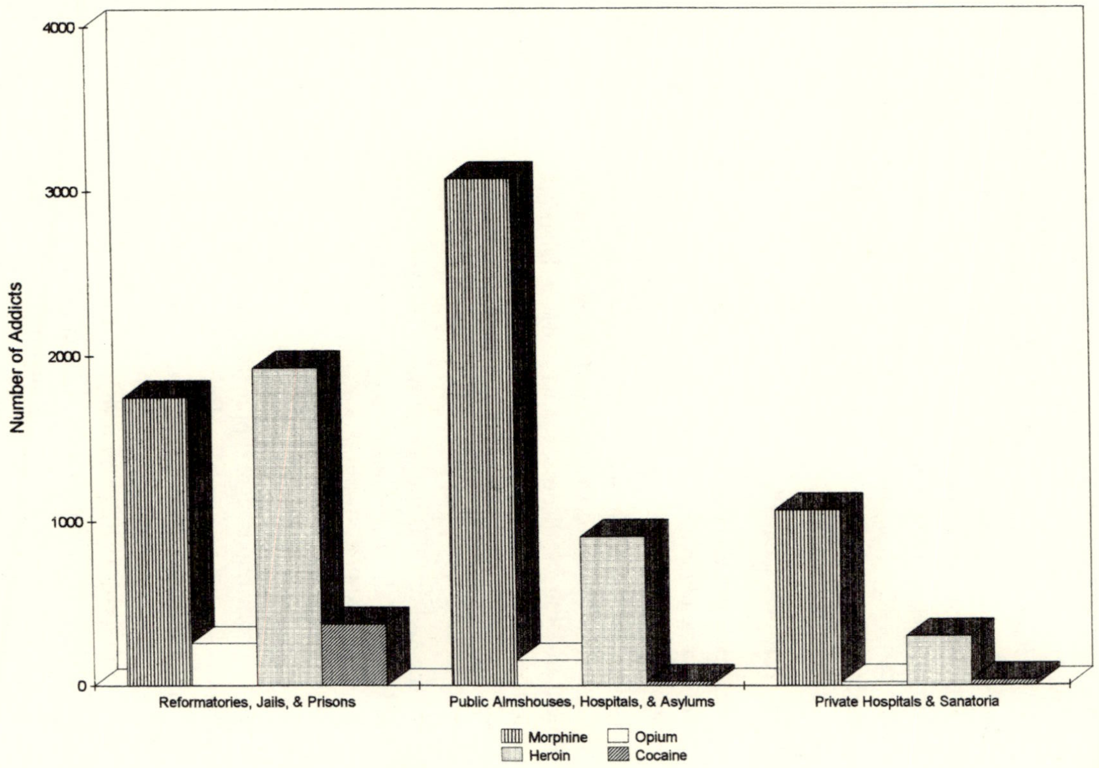

comparison between heroin addiction and leprosy (U.S. Senate, Committee on Printing 1924, 16–17). The metaphor stuck.

Those who have lived through the mid-to-late 1980s do not need to be reminded what happens when the public associates addictive drugs with crime sprees by slum dwellers. In 1920 the AMA's House of Delegates passed a resolution that heroin be eliminated from all medicines and that its importation, manufacture, and sale be banned in the United States. The measure was endorsed by police and penal authorities, and ultimately by Congress, which forbade the importation of opium to manufacture heroin in 1924. Stephen G. Porter, the bill's sponsor, hoped that other nations would emulate America's heroin ban, making it more difficult to divert the drug into the illicit traffic ("History of Heroin" 1953, 7; "Heroin and the International Conferences" 1953, 55–58; Musto 1987 [1973], 200–02).[11]

THE HEROIN COMPLEX

Yet within ten years of its prohibition, heroin was the mainstay of the illicit traffic practically everywhere in the United States. In the mid-to-late 1910s most heroin addicts lived (and died) in the New York–Philadelphia area. That was where most of the large heroin manufacturing and distribution companies were located and where diversion was therefore easiest, as when the American Drug Syndicate Company's Long Island plant was robbed of 150 pounds of heroin tablets in 1920. In other parts of the country, morphine or morphine-and-cocaine addicts were the norm (Courtwright 1982, 101–02; Jonnes 1996, 77).

By the end of 1920 the government had forbidden maintenance and had closed almost all of the municipal narcotic clinics. Some of the displaced patients were able to find doctors willing to write prescriptions. Those who suffered from chronic diseases like advanced tuberculosis, sympathetic figures in the eyes of both physicians and narcotic agents, had the most success in securing a continuous legal supply. But those who were "merely" addicted to narcotics—including virtually all heroin users—generally had to turn to the black market. Most black-market drugs were diverted from legitimate pharmaceutical manufacturers, who were making far more drugs than medically necessary during the 1920s. Enforcement of the Jones-Miller Act (1922) and a series of diplomatic agreements, culminating in the 1931 Limitation Convention to regulate international manufacturing, made diversion more difficult and brought licit production more into line with medical and scientific needs. Supplying the U.S. black market increasingly became a matter of smuggling and then distributing narcotics illicitly manufactured in such distant places as Turkey, the Balkans, and Shanghai.[12]

Heroin was the smuggler's drug par excellence. It was compact and potent, and did not spoil. It could be, and was, adulterated after arrival to increase profits. Even discounting for the adulteration, it was "cheaper for the amount of kick in it" (Helbrant 1941, 30).[13] Neophytes, wary of the needle, could sniff the drug. They could also afford it. Decks of adulterated heroin sold for as little as 50 cents apiece in Harlem during the Depression (Courtwright et al. 1989, 105).[14] These advantages made heroin the primary black-market narcotic throughout the United States, in fact throughout most of the world, by the mid-twentieth century ("History of Heroin," 7; D'Erlanger 1936, 94–95).

Not all addicts approved of the trend. American opium smokers, who regarded heroin as dangerous and déclassé, were especially upset. They would have continued as before, but their accustomed drug was becoming progressively scarcer and more expensive. They were victims of what the physician and anthropologist Joseph Westermeyer calls the pro-heroin effects of anti-opium laws. The rigorous enforcement of drug prohibition inevitably drives traffickers and users away from bulkier and more perishable narcotics like opium and toward heroin, with generally evil consequences (Westermeyer 1976, 1135–39).

Let me invoke the work of two other distinguished anthropologists, Vera Rubin and Lambros Comitas. They coined the phrase "ganja complex" to describe a particular pattern of chronic working-class cannabis use in Jamaica and other cultures (Rubin and Comitas 1975, ch. 4; Rubin 1975, 5–6). It seems to me that what had evolved in America by the 1930s was a distinctive "heroin complex." Its attributes can be summarized briefly. Most addicted users were male, poorly educated, irreligious, engaged in part- or full-time hustling; most lived in cities—about half in New York. Many female addicts were prostitutes. Initiated by sniffing, addicts switched to skin popping and mainlining to maximize the effect of adulterated heroin. They suffered high rates of morbidity, mortality, incarceration, and violence tied to disputes over drugs and money. They were part of a deviant, stratified subculture that revolved around the acquisition and use of heroin, had its own specialized language, and was at once mutually supportive and exploitative. "Never trust a junkie" was more than a prejudice of the straight world.

What happened to the heroin complex? Before World War II it was mostly white and, as social problems go, of modest significance. Harry Anslinger, longtime head of the Bureau of Narcotics, estimated that there were thirty-five thousand to fifty thousand nonmedical addicts in the country in 1938 (Anslinger 1938). By contrast, Joseph Greenwood, a Drug Enforcement Administration epidemiologist, estimated that there were 504,000 to 578,000 addicts (that is, a 95 percent confidence interval around an estimate of 546,000) in 1975 (Greenwood n.d.). Bearing in mind the critical things I and others have said about official prevalence estimates, there is still no question that the heroin complex of the 1930s was small-time compared with that of the 1970s or, for that matter, of the 1990s.

But before the heroin complex got larger, it got smaller. Addiction hit a record low during World War II. The country was prosperous. There was a sense of national purpose. Jobs were abundant and wages were high. Millions of susceptible youths joined the armed forces. There they might acquire the vices of smoking, drinking, and swearing, but not heroin using, at least not in the 1940s (Burnham 1993, 70–71, 101, 220–21). Back on the streets, prices were high and so was adulteration; black-market heroin was often only 1 percent pure by 1944, when it could be found at all.[15] Addicts had to boil down paregoric, eat *yen-shee* (the residue from smoking opium), bribe physicians, forge prescriptions, rob drugstores, switch to other drugs (such as barbiturates), or just plain quit (see Courtwright et al. 1989, 89, 107–08, 131, 168, 193–94, 268; "What's Cooking?" 1945, 99–100; U.S. Treasury Dept., Bureau of Narcotics 1945, 17; "History of Heroin," 8; and Maisel 1945). Some evidently stayed clean for the duration. Voluntary commitments of drug addicts in New York City, the nation's erstwhile heroin capital, dipped to almost zero by 1943 (Rosenthal 1951).

Heroin receded from the national consciousness during and immediately after the war. "In 1947 I was as innocent about drugs as I was about sex . . . ," William Styron wrote in his quasi-autobiographical *Sophie's Choice*. "Our present-day drug culture had not seen, that year, even the glimmerings of dawn, and my notion of addiction (if I had ever really thought of such a thing) was connected with the idea of 'dope fiends'—goggle-eyed madmen in straight jackets immured in backwater asylums, slavering molesters of children, zombies stalking the back streets of Chicago, comatose Chinese in their smoky dens, and so on. There was the taint about drugs of the irredeemably depraved, almost as evil as certain images of sexual intercourse—which until I was almost thirteen I visualized as a brutish act committed in secrecy upon dyed blondes by huge drunken unshaven ex-convicts with their shoes on. As for drugs, certainly I knew nothing about the types and subtle gradations of these substances" (Styron 1979, 311).

But then, in the late 1940s and early 1950s, the narcotic problem became more visible as the flow of smuggled heroin resumed (Jonnes 1996, chs. 8–10). The rituals of postwar addicts, the heroin complex, remained much the same. But their background was changing. They were now younger and darker-skinned. Just how many teenage addicts there were in the 1950s was much disputed. One of the more comprehensive studies, of newly reported addicts in New York State from 1952 to 1958, showed that about 19 percent were under twenty-one and just 5 percent under eighteen years of age (Schlesinger et al. 1959, 4389). Still, any teenage addiction was alarming, particularly in the apprehensive Cold War climate of the 1950s (see Campbell 2000).

Latino and, especially, black narcotic use was up sharply in the late 1940s and 1950s. From 1935 to 1947 only about 10 percent, on average, of those admitted to the Lexington and Fort Worth hospitals were black. By the mid-1950s the figure had risen to over 40 percent. "I saw a shift in the population," recalled one veteran of Lexington, who was readmitted in 1956. "They came mostly from Chicago and New York, the big cities. They used to say, 'Well, here comes a bunch on the chain from D.C.'—there were a lot of blacks from D.C. If you were arrested and brought there you were hooked up and chained, handcuffed to one another" (Courtwright et al. 1989, 15, quotation at 307).

Explanations for this dramatic development are various and politically sensitive. Some still cling to the "Godfather" conspiracy theory: the Mob decided to dump drugs in black neighborhoods. More plausible is Jill Jonnes's hepster role-model theory. When word got out that the coolest of the cool—black jazzmen like Charlie Parker—used heroin, scores of imitators, "conscientious objectors to the American Dream that never included them," quickly followed (Jonnes 1996, ch. 7, quotation at 121). This began a chain reaction. Older users initiated younger ones, who looked up to them. Dealers became admired figures. Bumpy Johnson, who dealt kilos and drove a Cadillac, was an "idol" to the author Claude Brown's generation, as were "other less well-known, neighborhood racketeers" (Brean 1951, 119; Brown 1984, 54). Brown, of course, grew up in Harlem. Underlying all of this was the shift of black population from the rural South, where heroin was practically non-existent, to the crowded urban slums, where the traffic was well established. Exposure matters.

The postwar revival of the heroin traffic, the involvement of organized crime (and, according to Anslinger, Communist China), the perceived spread of addiction among teenagers, and the very real spread of addiction in the barrios and ghettos contributed to a further hardening of narcotic policy. The outstanding feature of the 1951 Boggs Act, the 1956 Narcotic Control Act, and analogous state legislation ("Little Boggs Laws") was increasingly stiff mandatory minimum sentences. The 1956 statute even permitted juries to recommend the death penalty for those convicted of sales to minors, an indication of the symbolic importance of the endangered-youth issue.[16]

HEROIN AS THE CENTERPIECE OF AMERICA'S DRUG WARS

The events that followed 1956 properly belong to other contributors to this volume. I would, however, like to make one general observation about heroin's first century. Like any psychoactive drug that escapes the realm of healing for that of self-indulgence, heroin provoked a legislative response. What set heroin apart was the strength and persistence of that response.

By my count there were five, or perhaps four and a half, federal drug wars in the twentieth century. Heroin figured prominently in three of them. The first, longest, and most significant lasted from 1909 to about 1924. Driven by concerns about heroin and other narcotics, it resulted in the de facto criminalization of nonmedical addiction. The postwar expansion of the inner-city heroin complex triggered another major campaign in the 1950s, engineered by the Bureau of Narcotics and its congressional allies. Yet another heroin epidemic in the late 1960s gave rise to Nixon's drug war, a more enlightened and flexible undertaking than either its predecessors or its successor. Heroin was missing in action only in the marijuana skirmish of the mid-1930s and the Reagan-era drug war. The latter grew out of the increased use of marijuana and cocaine, especially in the form of crack. Though crack eclipsed heroin as drug enemy number one in the late 1980s, heroin made a slow but steady comeback during the 1990s, when increasing supplies and unprecedented levels of street purity provoked new concern. Once again, cocaine users, burned out and jittery, began turning to heroin, just as they had earlier in the century. While it seems unlikely that heroin will again completely supplant cocaine, as it did during the 1920s and 1930s, or will recover the black-market prominence that it enjoyed during the 1950s and 1960s, its suppression remains a critical object of American drug policy.

NOTES

1. "Questionaire [sic] re Drug Habit," Box 6, and Kolb to John Remig, 14 November 1927, Box 4, Kolb Papers. This was an almost universal judgment by the 1920s. William White, an authority on treatment history, adds that early twentieth-century proprietary drug cures of the mail-order variety almost never mentioned heroin in their advertising (personal communication).

2. The authoritative *Merck's 1907 Index* refers only to heroin's use as a "cough-sedative" and antispasmodic, recommended in cases of phthisis (tuberculosis), bronchitis, asthma, and so forth. For further discussion of the controversy surrounding heroin's use as an analgesic, see Courtwright 1982, 93. For more on early warnings, see Musto 1974, 176.

3. See the Heroin and Antikamnia brochures in the Antikamnia Chemical Company Collection. Similar items can be found in the Charles L. Mitchell Company Collection and the Lehn and Fink Collection. I am grateful to Charles Greifenstein for calling this material to my attention. See also Fiedler 1979, 59–72; and Haussmann 1891, 181–82.

4. Another interesting case involves Bromo-Seltzer, an over-the-counter preparation consisting of acetanilid, bromide, caffeine, and citric salts. In the 1930s

several deaths were attributed to the product, much to the discomfiture of its manufacturers and advertisers. It turned out, however, that the victims were using Bromo-Seltzer as an analgesic to cope with headaches and other painful symptoms arising from chronic diseases that were the real causes of their demise. Fifty years earlier, they probably would have been using opiates. (See J. Walter Thompson Archives, Forum Series, Emerson Drug Company, January 12, 1937.)

5. Leroy Street tells a version of the story in which the first users were Chinese "hopheads" arrested sometime during or after 1909 for attempting to secure smoking opium in defiance of the national import ban. "A lot of them had a bad cough; when they were in jail they gave them heroin, which is a *marvelous* cure for a cough. But aside from that, it's a hell of an addictive drug" (Courtwright et al. 1989, 289).

6. The date of the first heroin addiction case admitted to Bellevue also was 1910 (Bloedorn 1917, 312). In 1911 Harlow Brooks and H. R. Mixwell noted that "the habit is by no means infrequent especially on the extreme east and west sides of [New York City]" (Brooks and Mixwell 1911, 386). In short, all available historical evidence suggests that nonmedical heroin use took hold in New York City during or just before 1910 and expanded rapidly thereafter. The number of Bellevue heroin cases went from 1 in 1910 to 649 in 1916 (Bloedorn 1917, 312).

7. For national cigarette production figures, see Brecher et al. 1972, 230. For New York consumption, see Kluger 1996, 62. A study conducted by Sylvester Leahy showed a preponderance of children of immigrants ($n = 58$) over children of native-born parents ($n = 53$) among heroin addicts (Leahy 1915, 260).

8. Wiley 1917, 150. I am grateful to H. Wayne Morgan for calling this source to my attention.

9. The idea that tobacco leads to drunkenness and other vices has a long history. See, for example, Short 1750, 250; Rush 1798, 270; and Grimshaw 1853, 27–28.

10. Lawrence Kolb, the man fated to deal with America's narcotic obsessives, thought that these views couldn't be crazier. He diplomatically said so in his testimony at the same hearings (U. S. Senate, Committee on Printing 1924, 26–27). Nevertheless, the direct heroin-crime link pushed by Hobson and others affected public perception.

11. For a critical account of Porter's subsequent diplomatic maneuverings, see McAllister 2000, ch. 3.

12. Meyer and Parssinen (1998, chs. 1, 9) offer a comprehensive overview of international developments and how they impacted on the U.S. black market. For more on the 1931 convention as a watershed in international control efforts, see McAllister 2000, ch. 3. Global figures on the declining licit manufacture are found in "History of Heroin," 12.

13. William S. Burroughs, the "master addict" of his generation, was of the opinion that heroin was eight times as powerful as morphine (from letter to Allen Ginsberg in Burroughs 1993, 215).

14. In the 1920s decks reportedly sold for $1.00, $1.50, $2.00, $3.00, and $5.00 (New York State Commission on Prisons 1924).

15. Well before Pearl Harbor (December 1941), Anslinger had been stockpiling heroin as a strategic material, which drove up the price. The war itself brought tighter border controls, shipping disruptions, and travel restrictions. Seats on the remaining commercial airplanes, for example, were assigned on a priority basis to key government and military personnel. The term "VIP" was born of wartime flight rationing.

16. For more on postwar minority use and the federal laws of the 1950s, see Courtwright et al. 1989, 14–20; and Musto 1974, 230–32. The subject is also treated at length in the expanded edition of Courtwright 1982 (2001).

REFERENCES

Anslinger, Harry J. 1936. Memorandum to the Secretary of the Treasury. September 3. Vertical file "Heroin—History." Drug Enforcement Administration Library, Arlington, Va.

———. 1938. Memorandum and data sheet. March 16. Treasury Department File 0120-9, Record Group 170, National Archives II. College Park, Md.

Antikamnia Chemical Company Collection. Medical Trade Ephemera. College of Physicians of Philadelphia Library.

Bailey, Pearce. 1916. "The Heroin Habit." New Republic 6 (April 22): 314–16.

Blanchard, R. M. 1913. "Heroin and Soldiers." Military Surgeon 33.

Bloedorn, W. A. 1917. "Studies of Drug Addiction." U. S. Naval Medical Bulletin 11.

Brean, Herbert. 1951. "Children in Peril." Life. June 11.

Brecher, Edward M., et al. 1972. Licit and Illicit Drugs. Boston: Little, Brown.

Brooks, Harlow, and H. R. Mixwell. 1911. "Two Cases of Heroin Habituation." New York State Journal of Medicine 11.

Brown, Claude. 1984. "Manchild in Harlem." New York Times Magazine. September 16.

Burnham, John. 1993. Bad Habits: Drinking, Smoking, Taking Drugs, Gambling, Sexual Misbehavior, and Swearing in American History. New York: New York University Press.

Burroughs, William S. 1993. The Letters of William S. Burroughs, 1945–1959. Edited by Oliver Harris. New York: Viking Press.

Campbell, Nancy D. 2000. Using Women: Gender, Drug Policy, and Social Justice. New York: Routledge.

"Caution Regarding Heroin." 1900. Druggists Circular and Chemical Gazette 44 (March): 44.

Charles L. Mitchell Company Collection. Medical Trade Ephemera. College of Physicians of Philadelphia Library.

Chase, J. Frank, et al. 1912. The Dope Evil. Boston: New England Watch and Ward Society.

Courtwright, David T. 1982. Dark Paradise: Opiate Addiction in America Before 1940. Cambridge, Mass.: Harvard University Press. Enlarged ed. 2001.

Courtwright, David, Herman Joseph, and Don Des Jarlais. 1989. Addicts Who Survived: An Oral History of Narcotic Use in America, 1923–1965. Knoxville: University of Tennessee Press.

D'Erlanger, Baron Harry. 1936. *The Last Plague of Egypt*. London: Lovat Dickson and Thompson.

Farr, Clifford B. 1915. "The Relative Frequency of the Morphine and Heroin Habits: Based upon Some Observations at the Philadelphia General Hospital." *New York Medical Journal* 101.

Fiedler, William C. 1979. "Antikamnia: The Story of a Pseudo-Ethical Pharmeutical." *Pharmacy in History* 21.

Floret, [Theobald]. 1898. "Klinische Versuche über die Wirkung und Anwendung des Heroins." *Therapeutische Monatshefte* 12.

Greenwood, Joseph A. n.d. TS memorandum, "Estimated Drug Abusers, Estimated Addicts, 1969–1975." Vertical File, "Addiction—Incidence, 1973–1975." Drug Enforcement Administration Library, Arlington, Virginia.

Grimshaw, A. H. 1853. *An Essay on the Physical and Moral Effects of the Use of Tobacco as a Luxury*. New York: William Howard.

Haussmann, F. W. 1891. "Antikamnia." *American Journal of Pharmacy* 63.

Helbrant, Maurice. 1941. *Narcotic Agent*. New York: Vanguard.

"Heroin and the International Conferences on Narcotics of 1925 and 1931." 1953. *Bulletin on Narcotics* 5.

"Heroin Hydrochloride." 1906. JAMA 47.

"History of Heroin." 1953. *Bulletin on Narcotics* 5.

Jonnes, Jill. 1996. *Hep-Cats, Narcs, and Pipe Dreams: A History of America's Romance with Illegal Drugs*. New York: Scribner.

J. Walter Thompson Company Archives. Forum Series. Emerson Drug Company. January 12 1937. Special Collections Library. Duke University.

Kane, Francis Fisher, et al. 1917. "Drugs and Crime: Report of Committee 'G' of the Institute." *Journal of the American Institute of Criminal Law and Criminology* 8.

Kluger, Richard. 1996. *Ashes to Ashes: America's Hundred-Year Cigarette War, the Public Health, and the Unabashed Triumph of Philip Morris*. New York: Knopf.

Kolb Papers. National Library of Medicine. Bethesda, Md.

Leahy, Sylvester. 1915. "Some Observations on Heroin Habitués." *Psychiatric Bulletin of the New York State Hospitals* n.s. 8.

Lehn and Fink Collection. Medical Trade Ephemera. College of Physicians of Philadelphia Library.

McAllister, William B. 2000. *Drug Diplomacy in the Twentieth Century: An International History*. London: Routledge.

McIver, Joseph, and George E. Price. 1916. "Drug Addiction." JAMA 66.

McTavish, Jan R. 1987. "Aspirin in Germany: The Pharmaceutical Industry and the Pharmaceutical Profession." *Pharmacy in History* 29.

McWilliams, John C. 1990. *The Protectors: Harry J. Anslinger and the Federal Bureau of Narcotics, 1930–1962*. Newark: University of Delaware Press.

Maisel, Albert Q. 1945. "Getting the Drop on Dope." *Liberty*. November 24.

Manges, Morris. 1898. "The Treatment of Coughs with Heroin." *New York Medical Journal* 68.

———. 1900. "A Second Report on the Therapeutics of Heroin." *New York Medical Journal* 71.

Meyer, Kathryn, and Terry Parssinen. 1998. *Webs of Smoke: Smugglers, Warlords, Spies, and the History of the International Drug Trade*. Lanham, Md.: Rowman and Littlefield.

Musto, David F. 1974. "Early History of Heroin in the United States." In *Addiction*. Edited by Peter G. Bourne. New York: Academic Press.

———. 1987 [1973]. *The American Disease: Origins of Narcotic Control*. Enl. ed. New York: Oxford University Press.

———. 1990. "Illicit Price of Cocaine in Two Eras: 1908–14 and 1982–89." *Connecticut Medicine 54*.

New York State, Narcotic Drug Control Commission. 1920. *Second Annual Report*. Edited by Walter R. Herrick. Albany: J. B. Lyon.

New York State Commission on Prisons. Special Report on Drug Addiction. Vertical File, "Addiction—Incidence [to] 1959." Drug Enforcement Administration Library. Arlington, Virginia.

Pettey, George E. 1903. "The Heroin Habit: Another Curse." *Alabama Medical Journal* 15: 174–80.

Rosenthal, Herbert C. 1951. "How Much of a Menace Is the Drug Menace?" *Pageant*. October.

Rubin, Vera, ed. 1975. *Cannabis and Culture*. The Hague: Mouton.

Rubin, Vera, and Lambros Comitas. 1975. *Ganja in Jamaica: A Medical Anthropological Study of Chronic Marijuana Use*. The Hague: Mouton.

Rush, Benjamin. 1798. *Essays: Literary, Moral and Philosophical*. Philadelphia: Thomas and Samuel F. Branford.

Scheffel, Carl. 1918. "The Etiology of Fifty Cases of Drug Addictions." *Medical Record* 94.

Schlesinger, Edward R., et al. 1959. "Experience with Reporting of Habitual Users of Narcotic Drugs in New York State." *New York State Journal of Medicine* 59.

Short, Thomas. 1750. *Discourses on Tea, Sugar, Milk-Made Wines, Spirits, Punch, Tobacco, etc.* London: T. Longman and A. Millar.

Spillane, Joseph F. 2000. *Cocaine: From Medical Marvel to Modern Menace in the United States, 1884–1920*. Baltimore: Johns Hopkins University Press.

Stokes, Charles F. 1918. "The Problem of Narcotic Addiction of Today." *Medical Record* 93.

Street, Leroy, with David Loth. 1953. *I Was a Drug Addict*. New York: Random House.

Styron, William. 1979. *Sophie's Choice*. New York: Random House.

Symposium "'The Doctor and the Drug Addict.'" 1920. JAMA 75.

Towns, Charles B. 1916. *Habits That Handicap: The Menace of Opium, Alcohol, and Tobacco, and the Remedy*. New York: Century.

Tuttle, Charles H. n.d. Memorandum to the National Commission on Law Observance and Enforcement. Box 56. Richmond C. Hobson Papers. Library of Congress.

U. S. Senate, Committee on Printing. 1924. *Hearing . . . on a Resolution to Print Fifty Million Additional Copies of an Article Entitled "The Peril of Narcotic Drugs"* . . . 3 June 1924. Washington, D.C.: U.S. Government Printing Office.

U.S. Treasury Department. 1919. *Traffic in Narcotic Drugs: Report of Special Committee of Investigation Appointed March 25, 1918, by the Secretary of the Treasury.* Washington, D. C.: U.S. Government Printing Office.

U.S. Treasury Department, Bureau of Narcotics. 1945. *Traffic in Opium and Other Dangerous Drugs for the Year Ended December 31, 1944.* Washington, D.C.: U.S. Government Printing Office.

Westermeyer, Joseph. 1976. "The Pro-Heroin Effects of Anti-Opium Laws in Asia." *Archives of General Psychiatry* 33.

"What's Cooking?" 1945. *Newsweek.* April 9.

W. H. Schieffelin and Company Collection. Medical Trade Ephemera. College of Physicians of Philadelphia Library.

Wiley, Harvey W. 1917. "The Alcohol and Drug Habit and Its Prophylaxis." *Proceedings of the Second Pan American Scientific Congress,* vol. 9. Washington, D.C.: U.S. Government Printing Office.

Wolff, Paul. 1932. "Drug Addiction—A World-Wide Problem." JAMA 98.

Wood, Horatio C., Jr. 1899. "The Newer Substitutes for Morphine." *Merck's Archives* 1.

Part II

Inside Policymaking

2

One Hundred Years of Heroics

Daniel Patrick Moynihan

On May 1, 1898, Admiral Dewey triumphed in the Battle of Manila Bay. The United States seized the Philippines, became an imperial power, and shortly thereafter commenced a crusade against opium, first in the new colony, next in China itself. In time the crusade would reach our shores.

Three months and one day following the battle—on August 2, 1898—the Bayer Pharmaceutical Company of Elberfeld, Germany, obtained a U.S. trademark, no. 31,836, for a new cough medicine, a derivative of opium, called *heroin*. Tested on Bayer employees, the drug made them feel "heroisch." At that time, tuberculosis and pneumonia were the two leading causes of death in the United States. Both diseases provoked agonizing coughing, and the new drug promised relief. It was surely welcome. For a time.

On September 10, 1998, a century later, the Senate Committee on Finance met to approve the tariff legislation for the 105th Congress. Tariffs were once the principal source of revenue for the federal government. Having amended the Constitution in 1913, we now rely on the income and payroll taxes for most federal revenue, but tariff schedules and the Customs Service still are of great importance to international trade.

This being technically a revenue bill, it had come from the House of Representatives as H.R. 3809, the "Drug Free Borders Act of 1998." And indeed the House bill, the Senate bill, and most emphatically the testimony that had preceded them put the greatest emphasis on drug smuggling and drug seizures, with graphic accounts by Treasury officials (the Customs Service is part of the Treasury Department) of the latest successes of Operation Hard Line along our southwestern border. They reported 33,000 pounds of cocaine, 600,000 pounds of marijuana, and 190 pounds of heroin seized in just the previous fiscal year. Next, the triumphs of Operation Gateway, directed against the "air and maritime threat in Puerto Rico, the Virgin Islands, and their surrounding waters" (18,000 pounds of cocaine, 80 pounds of heroin). In all, customs agents seized some 2,444 pounds of heroin in fiscal year 1997 (Kelly and Johnson 1998).

At about this time, General Barry R. McCaffrey reported that in 1997 U.S. border inspectors had searched a million or so trucks and railroad cars entering the United States from Mexico. Cocaine was discovered in six; heroin, presumably, about as often. Notwithstanding, on September 16, 1998, the House passed H.R. 4300, the Western Hemisphere Drug Elimination Act, by a vote of 384–39. The bill called for an 80 percent cut in the flow of illicit drugs into the United States by 2001, allocating an extra $2.6 billion to bring it off. Impossible, said the general, but with little evident impact.

What a distance we have come from the enthusiasms of the Progressive Era at the beginning of the century, when the United States undertook to persuade the great powers to keep opium out of Asia, culminating in the First International Conference on Opium in 1911, at The Hague. There was a second conference in 1913. The third occurred in 1914, concluding, as David F. Musto records, "three days before the assassination of Archduke Ferdinand" (Musto 1973 [1987], 53). There also was, of course, the inconvenient problem of addiction to narcotics here at home, where heroin (the "Sedative for Coughs") was legal and essentially unregulated.[1]

After sorting out the constitutional issue of separation of powers between the federal and state governments, Congress passed the Harrison Narcotic Act, reported first from the House Committee on Ways and Means, then from the Senate Committee on Finance. President Wilson signed the bill into law on December 17, 1914—fifteen months after the bill's sponsor, New York Representative Francis Burton Harrison, a Yale graduate and Tammany Democrat, resigned his seat to become Governor-General of the Philippines. What had begun as an "American crusade" to save the heathen, and just possibly enhance our exports, ended with our having to face our own narcotics problem, for indeed heroin and cocaine use had become epidemic in the first decade of the century. And now, a century later, we are still at it.

Let this be my theme. In the course of the nineteenth century the development of organic chemistry, principally in Germany, gave rise to a number of new drugs intended for medical use. The legal *prescription* of some of these led to a significant rate of iatrogenic addiction. Whereupon they were *proscribed*. But their illegal use continued, following epidemic cycles. For the most part, illegal drug use came to be defined as a law enforcement problem. Where it remains.

David Musto calculates that our first drug epidemic peaked between 1900 and World War I (Musto 1998). It thereupon subsided, owing in part, I should conjecture, to the Harrison Act. Domestic pharmaceutical production ceased, and foreign sources were slow to develop. I have an anecdote by way of evidence. I attended Benjamin Franklin High School in Manhattan in the years just before and just after our entry into World War II. Our original building was on East 108th Street, just off the original Puerto Rican neighborhood known as the barrio. Later, we moved to a new building, Mayor LaGuardia's pride, at 115th Street and York Avenue, in the area known as East Harlem. These were peaceable, stable, busy neighborhoods. Doubtless there was some crime; possibly there were some drugs; one never heard of either. Young people in our mid-teens, that is: we didn't hear. We were proud of our new school building and our extraordinary faculty. Indeed, my school day typically started at the New York Central Railroad's Harlem Station at 125th Street and Park Avenue. I would wait there until the appointed hour at which a beloved economics teacher would descend from his commuter train, and off we would go, propounding all the way. There was not the least sign of social disorder in 1942.

Now let us fast-forward, in truth not all that forward, to 1960. Vincent P. Dole, then a laboratory-based researcher at Rockefeller University, commuted to New York City from his home in Westchester. He recalled in a splendid lecture in 1991, "Addiction as a Public Health Problem," how he would mostly read or edit papers while he commuted, but at other times, otherwise:

> Occasionally, to save time in the morning, I left the train at the 125th Street Harlem Station and continued the trip to my laboratory on the elevated Third Avenue trolley (now gone). Walking the short distance between stations on 125th Street and then traveling 60 blocks on the elevated—in effect a moving aerial platform—I saw drugs being sold on the sidewalks, drunks sleeping in doorways, young men idling on corners, young women apparently available at a price, shabby buildings, and busy bars. (Dole 1991, 749)

This at the very same station where I had waited for my high school economics teacher eighteen years earlier.

In the 1950s I was an aide to Averell Harriman, who was then governor of New York. At that time mental illness was thought to be our principal public health problem, and during those years we commenced the use of tranquilizers in our mental institutions, with important if unanticipated consequences in the form of deinstitutionalization. This was the work of Paul Hoch, a great psychiatrist. But illicit drugs a public health problem? Nothing one heard of. In 1961 I moved to Washington and became a member of the sub-cabinet of President John F. Kennedy. In time, I would be much involved in the development of the War on Poverty, as Lyndon Johnson called it. There were surely many problems out there. But drugs? Again, nothing we'd heard of. Perhaps if we had known more about juvenile delinquency, we would have come upon the subject. But, if it was there, we missed it.

I left government in 1965, and returned four years later in 1969 as Assistant to the President for Urban Affairs. In that brief interval our cities had exploded in rioting and a devastating heroin epidemic had broken out, with epicenters in our central cities.

Looking back, I note that the urban riots ended almost as abruptly as they had begun. Some decades later there would be random convulsions, but nothing like the summer upheavals that many thought had become a fixed pattern of American civic life. Drawing on the work of Edward C. Banfield and Lloyd E. Ohlin, I was of the view that rioting is aversive behavior, not fun for long, nor readily repeated.

In the White House I set forth a version of urban triage. A hot line was installed in the basement. Frantic calls would come in. This or that metropolis was about to "blow." This had become a form of threat behavior. The alarming news was typically accompanied by the suggestion that this grant or that appointment might just prevent disaster. We would ask, Is the explosion otherwise inevitable? Absolutely, would come the reply. Then, we would say, we were sorry, that resources were limited, that we were sending grants or appointments only to places where there was still hope. Typically, in time, another call would arrive reporting that things were looking up in the previously doomed city and that a grant might lock the progress in.

Now, clearly, this bit of theater could have had little effect in itself. But riots are aversive and they *did* stop. The heroin epidemic, however, only got worse, and urban disorder became endemic. Thus, early in the Nixon administration, a group of eminent Washingtonians—civic persons, important people—asked me to ask if the President might garrison the capital, such was the outbreak of crime and what might be called low-level violence.[2] Some of this, surely, reflected the huge demographic bulge of persons fifteen to twenty-five years of age in that decade. (To get a bit ahead of my story, when I left the Nixon administration, I became a member of the President's Science Advisory Committee. James S. Coleman formed a small group to look into this. We soon discovered, if that is the term, that the bulge had passed. In 1973 I could give a lecture titled "Peace," stating that the days of campus upheaval were behind us, as the baby boomers had moved on—to Wall Street, for the most part [Moynihan 1973].)

But while the riots and upheavals dissipated, as I remarked, heroin stayed, and the new administration had only the faintest idea of what, if anything, could be done. Certainly I had none.

David Musto has found in the National Archives a six-page memorandum for the Attorney General that I wrote on February 11, 1969, twenty days or so after the new President's inauguration (Moynihan 1969a). It draws heavily on conversations I had been having with James Q. Wilson at Harvard, and could be said to reflect the faint beginnings of a new federal strategy in crime control. My first point was succinct: "Organized crime exists because of laws prohibiting the consumption of certain goods and services for which there is in fact a large demand." Thomas C. Schelling, I continued, had shown that "the effect of these prohibitions is to grant the criminal the position of a manufacturer protected by a huge tariff: . . . a quasi-monopolistic position." This was the supply side. I went on to discuss the possibility of demand reduction, "for example the provision of methadone to heroin addicts—methadone is in effect a drug that can be bought on the open market."

Then: "It is time for a major inquiry into the subject of heroin addiction, and also for serious foreign policy initiatives to cut down the smuggling." I was alarmist: "We are at the point . . . where the consequences of heroin addiction are threatening the social stability of the nation." I allowed that "academic lore" had it that "most of the heroin brought into the East Coast is grown in Turkey and Syria, and processed in France." (I should have said "opium," but such was the state of our knowledge at the time.) We should find out.

I then went on to adumbrate one of the great contributions Jim Wilson has made to social science and society: "Wilson . . . feels that a dramatic, visible, openly experimental effort to cut down street crime in the worst precinct of, say, the ten largest cities in the nation might very well . . . [teach us something]."

Thus we see the beginnings of the "broken window theory" which he and George L. Kelling set forth in the *Atlantic Monthly* in 1982 and which has been so widely adopted recently as a police strategy (Wilson and Kelling 1982, 1092). It also, of course, fits in nicely with Norman E. Zinberg's triad, "drug, set, and setting" (Zinberg 1984). If you live in a neighborhood in which illicit drugs are *not* for sale on street corners—well, you might just quit the stuff, or maybe never even start.

The memorandum to the Attorney General produced a measure of interest in the new administration, especially with regard to the Turkish and French involvement—an echo, perhaps, of our earnest initiatives abroad at the outset of the century. But with perhaps a touch more realism, at least on the part of some. Not me. In August 1969, now a member of the Cabinet, I slipped out of the country heading for India, then Istanbul, then Paris. I met with the appropriate officials, offered assistance to the Turks, invoked the Marshall Plan to the French, and returned with the rudiments of an agreement, which Egil Krogh would later formalize and implement, to put an end to farm-by-farm opium production in Turkey and heroin production in France.

As I have related elsewhere, upon my return I found myself in a helicopter with George P. Shultz heading from Camp David. I told him of my triumph. He looked up from his papers and nodded. "No," I came back, "this is really BIG." Same response. More than a little deflated, I pondered for a moment, and then suggested that what he was thinking was that as long as there is a demand, there will be a supply. Whereupon that great statesman and sometime professor of economics at the University of Chicago looked up from his papers, smiled approvingly, and said, "You know, there is hope for you yet."

Indeed, hope was abroad in the Nixon administration at this time. We knew nothing much of this subject—but neither had the administrations of Theodore Roosevelt, Taft, or Wilson—but it was fair to think we might learn. President Nixon put drug abuse on the national agenda in a way it had not been for a half-century and more. In December 1969 the Governors' Conference met in Washington to consider the subject. I was asked to give the luncheon address at the Department of State. I took as my theme "The Whiskey Culture and the Drug Culture," contending that early on in our national existence we had had considerable problems with the first, and now we were dealing with the second. There was a continuity:

> Let me offer one general idea. Drug use—and abuse—represents simply one more instance of the impact of technology on society. This is the central experience of modern society. At one or two removes, most of the ills we suffer are the consequences of technology. . . . From nuclear weapons to cyclamates, this is what is so unsettling about modern life. . . . But for the moment one of the tasks of government is to keep technology from rending the fabric of society.

I spoke as one with a limited view of the capacity of government to alter behavior:

> We were not able to prevent the use of alcohol, and we have not been able to bring it under social control for millions of our people. This seems to me to be a fact to be reckoned with. I am always impressed when I come upon a problem which others have tried to solve and have failed to solve, particularly when this has involved government efforts. I prefer not to assume that the others were simply stupid, or venal, or uninterested. I prefer to assume it is a tough problem.
>
> So also, obviously, is the problem of drug use. We have had drug prohibition for fifty-five years now. And here we are at this conference. Not exactly a record of success. . . .

On further thought, it will be seen that we know one other thing. *There is not going to be any cheap way out of this.* (Moynihan 1969b)

In December 1992 I was invited to give the inaugural Norman E. Zinberg lecture at the John F. Kennedy School of Government. I called the lecture "Iatrogenic Government: Social Policy and Drug Research" (Moynihan 1992). I made the argument that in dealing with drugs, "we are required to choose between a crime problem and a public health problem. In choosing to prohibit drugs, we choose to have a more or less localized—but ultimately devastating—crime problem rather than a mental health problem." Devastating indeed. In 1980 there were some twenty-four thousand inmates in state and federal prisons jailed for drug law violations—7 percent of the inmate population. By 1996 there were well over a quarter-million (287,194) state and federal inmates jailed for drug law violations—24 percent of the inmate population, which had grown to 1.2 million. In a decade and a half, while the nation's adult population grew by 19 percent, the number of state and federal inmates jailed for drug law violations grew by over 1,100 percent (CASA 1997).

These numbers, astonishing as they are, understate the situation. In January 1998 the National Center on Addiction and Substance Abuse at Columbia University released a report, *Behind Bars: Substance Abuse and America's Prison Population* (CASA 1997), which estimates that substance abuse and addiction have shaped the lives of 80 percent of our prison and local jail population. (That population—1.7 million, including persons held in local jails—is larger than our fourth largest city, Houston.) According to the report:

Eighty-one percent of the 1,076,625 state inmates, 80 percent of the 105,544 Federal inmates, and 77 percent of the 518,492 local jail inmates violated drug or alcohol laws, were high at the time they committed their crimes, stole property to buy drugs, or have a history of drug and alcohol abuse and addiction—or share some combination of these characteristics. (CASA 1997)

Within a few years, should current trends continue, we will be spending $100 million a day to jail individuals with serious drug and alcohol problems.

These dreary data follow enactment, prompted by the "crack" cocaine epidemic that struck in the mid-1980s, of the most ambitious drug control legislation Congress ever has passed, the Anti-Drug Abuse Act of 1988. The crack epidemic roared up from the Caribbean like one of those tropical hurricanes, wreaking all manner of havoc. Anticipated but not prepared for. I was familiar with the work of David Allen and had read the paper he and others had written for *Lancet*, "Epidemic Free-Base Cocaine Abuse: Case Study from the Bahamas" (Jeckel et al. 1986). The New York City Police

Department had spotted it right off. But our Centers for Disease Control scarcely noticed it. Somehow we just don't get this subject.

Of necessity Congress did: the public demanded action. Something, anything. In May 1988 Majority Leader Robert C. Byrd of West Virginia appointed Senator Sam Nunn of Georgia and me cochairmen of the Democratic Substance Abuse Working Group and charged us with developing a proposal for drug control legislation by the end of June. That is, in a hurry. Minority Leader Robert J. Dole of Kansas appointed Republicans to a similar task force. We set to work in a bipartisan manner.

We met our deadline, June 29, 1988, and issued a somber report:

> Drug use among youth is an index [of trouble]. Widespread drug use appeared suddenly in the 1960's and has increased to epidemic levels, mutating as epidemics do. (The National Commission on Marijuana and Drug Abuse of 1972–73 hardly mentioned cocaine.) While heroin use ravaged slums, LSD plagued prep schools. Cocaine, a drug of fashion in the 1970's, has mutated to "crack." It is roaring across the ghettos, spreading into the most prosperous neighborhoods, making its way back upwards in the social hierarchy. Age of initiation declines. Health impairment rises. The statistics are well enough known, but new findings focus on the increasing number of children *born* with drug-related disease or impairment. . . .
>
> The 1985 National Household Survey on Drug Abuse gives us a good look at the numbers. Some 23 million Americans had used illicit drugs in the previous 30 days. But use is concentrated among youth: 15.1 percent of those 12 to 17 years of age and 25.5 percent of those 18 to 25 were users.
>
> We are talking about our future, and there is a shadow over it. Young people everywhere are endangered, but most viciously, virulently, the young people of the inner cities. The violence associated with drug use could drastically alter American society. Single-parent families could become no-parent families: a devastating prospect already taking shape. (Moynihan and Nunn 1988)

From the outset, knowing that supply interdiction during the Nixon era was at most a brief success (after we ended the "French Connection," opium and heroin production merely moved elsewhere), I argued—quietly, so as not to disturb the public peace—that any new legislation must focus on demand reduction. That is, the user. We were able, at least for a while, to achieve some degree of consensus: the notion was that 60 percent of funding under our new bill would be earmarked for demand-reduction activities; the remaining 40 percent would be for supply reduction. I remarked on the floor of the Senate during consideration of the bill that

> We have set forth the principle of treatment on request [treatment on demand sounded too imperious]. We have set forth the principle that when you are in an epidemic you do not close your hospitals. . . .

In the end, the overwhelming challenge is that of medical care, treatment, and discovery. . . . [W]e have 70 million Americans who have used illicit drugs, and a good 7 million for whom it is an immediate, pressing problem today, as it was yesterday and will be tomorrow. . . .

Obviously we cannot put 7 million Americans in prison, or if we did we would not be the country we are today. And they do not need to be in prison. They need to be set free from their addiction which they have acquired in the manner that epidemic diseases are acquired: in their environment. . . .

If this were more of a middle-class disease, there would be more response. Right now in its epidemic mode as crack addiction, it is a disease of the slums. But diseases do not stay in slums. . . . Mr. President, they break out. They have done so through history. And this one will also, partly because it is so easy as a disease to contract. (*Congressional Record* 1988)

Democratic and Republican task forces were also established in the House. We acted with dispatch and passed a bill on October 22, 1988, the last bill of the 100th Congress. It became law in November, as the Anti-Drug Abuse Act of 1988 (P.L. 100–690). But as the bill made its way through House and Senate deliberations and quasi-conference committee negotiations, its emphasis shifted incrementally from demand reduction to supply reduction and, especially, to law enforcement. I suppose this was inevitable. Fear of crime far outstripped concern for addicts. And, just a few weeks away from the 1988 elections, it was inevitable that members of one party, then in the minority, would offer a steady stream of law enforcement amendments—a federal death penalty for "drug kingpins" and such—designed to make the other party look "soft" on crime. In the end, the bill authorized some $2.7 billion yearly in anti-drug activities. The deal had been a 60–40 ratio in favor of demand reduction; in the end it was the other way around. Now the ratio is about 2:1.

There were warning signs. The Anti-Drug Abuse Act of 1988 stated: "It is the declared policy of the United States Government to create a Drug-Free America by 1995" (P.L. 100–690, Subtitle F [Sec. 5251]). A war to be won in seven years. You need the military for that. We established the Office of National Drug Control Policy in the Executive Office of the President. It was headed by a so-called czar and included a Deputy Director for Demand Reduction and, listed next in the legislation, a Deputy Director for Supply Reduction. But, over the years, czars came and went. Our forceful first director, William Bennett, was followed by a political appointee with no apparent views on the subject. Deputy directors departed. No one has matched Dr. Herbert D. Kleber, who came down from Yale and served as the first Deputy Director for Demand Reduction for two years. The position is vacant *now*!

At a November 1997 NIDA-National Institute of Justice conference, "The Crack Decade: Research Perspectives and Lessons Learned," David Musto noted, "Research into the biological mechanisms of addiction appears to rise and fall depending on the public's anxiety level over drugs and whether the medical/therapeutic approach is in vogue. In the first epidemic, medical treatment approaches eventually gave way to an almost exclusive reliance on law enforcement and sustained scientific research fell precipitously" (Musto 1997). The pattern repeats.

Despite the fact that "funding for treatment of substance abuse has been a bipartisan failure," as Herbert Kleber put it a few years ago, knowledge *is* edging on. We have learned much over the years about "drug, set, and setting." Or, should I say, those who are research scientists, treatment providers, sociologists, and criminologists have done.

We in Congress still talk about the "war on drugs." In that 1969 address to the Governors' Conference, I stated:

> Technology has unleashed an enormous social agent which threatens us in the most serious way. The humility with which we approach this problem will almost be a measure of the maturity and responsibility with which we do so. It is easy enough to fail in these efforts: it will take moral courage and intellectual stamina to succeed. (Moynihan 1969b)

Nearly thirty years later, I feel even more humility is needed. But in Congress this is a minority view. Not long ago I received a letter from eight of my colleagues urging me to cosponsor the Western Hemisphere Drug Elimination Act of 1998, the bill I mentioned earlier, to "restore a *balanced* drug control strategy by renewing our commitment to international eradication and interdiction." In the face of a century of finding, this won't happen. Or consider—and I mean no disrespect here—former House Speaker Newt Gingrich's reaction to the Clinton administration's proposal for a ten-year drug control strategy, as David Musto recounts in a *Washington Post* article:

> The Speaker of the House rejected the strategy's goal as too drawn out and defeatist. . . . Newt Gingrich feels that a 10-year strategy indicates pessimism and perhaps lassitude in dealing with the drug problem. The Civil War, he says, "took just four years to save the Union and abolish slavery." Why can't we solve the drug problem, another form of slavery, in just a few years?

Musto goes on:

> Demanding quick solutions to the drug problem inevitably leads to frustration. . . . This may lead to more severe penalties, the scapegoating of minorities and, finally, discouragement. . . . Promises of a quick fix may energize concerned citizens for a while, but the larger effect is to discourage them. Repeated, hyped, short-term drug campaigns to end drug abuse "once and for all" (a federal government slogan of 1972) are reminiscent of cocaine abuse: Every time the same

dose is taken the impact lessens, the temptation to increase the dose escalates and, finally, you have burnout. (Musto 1998)

You have to be careful about what you do, what you promise.

I would, however, conclude on an optimistic note. Mildly optimistic. Let me share with you a cautionary tale, instructive of what is possible and also what we ought to be aware of. I remarked earlier that I was in the Harriman administration in New York in the 1950s. Early in 1955, Harriman met with his new Commissioner of Mental Hygiene, Paul Hoch, who described the development of a tranquilizer called reserpine, derived from *Rauwolfia serpentina*, at one of the state's mental hospitals. The medication had been clinically tested and appeared to be an effective treatment for many severely psychotic patients, increasing the percentage of patients discharged. Dr. Hoch recommended that it be used systemwide; Harriman found the money.

That same year Congress created the Joint Commission on Mental Health and Illness with a view to formulating "comprehensive and realistic recommendations" in this area, which was then a matter of considerable public concern. Year after year the population of mental institutions grew; year after year new facilities had to be built. Ballot measures to approve the issuance of general obligation bonds for building the facilities appeared in just about every election. Or so it seemed.

The discovery of tranquilizers was adventitious. Physicians were seeking cures for disorders they were just beginning to understand. Even a limited success made it possible to believe that the incidence of this particular range of disorders, which had seemingly required persons to be confined against their will or even awareness, could be greatly reduced. The congressional commission submitted its report in 1961; it was seen to propose a nationwide program of deinstitutionalization.

Late in 1961, President Kennedy appointed an interagency committee to prepare legislative recommendations based on the report. I represented Secretary of Labor Arthur J. Goldberg on this committee and drafted its final submission. This included the recommendation of the National Institute of Mental Health that two thousand "community mental health centers" (one for every hundred thousand people) be built by 1980. A buoyant presidential message to Congress followed, early in 1963. "If we apply our medical knowledge and social insights fully," President Kennedy stated, "all but a small portion of the mentally ill can eventually achieve a wholesome and a constructive social adjustment." A "concerted national attack on mental disorders [was] now possible and practical" (Kennedy 1963, 129). The President signed the Community Mental Health Centers Construction Act on October 31, 1963—his last public bill-signing ceremony (Kennedy 1963, 825). He gave me a pen.

The mental hospitals emptied out. The number of patients in state and county mental hospitals peaked in 1955 at 558,922 and has declined every year since then, to 61,722 in 1996. But we never came near to building the two thousand community mental health centers. Only some 482 received federal construction funds from 1963 to 1980. The next year, 1981, the program was folded into the Alcohol, Drug Abuse, and Mental Health block grant program, where it disappeared from view.

Even when centers *were* built, the results were hardly as hoped for. David Musto has noted that the planners had bet on improving national mental health "by improving the quality of general community life through *expert knowledge*, not merely by more effective treatment of the already ill" (Musto 1975, 67; my emphasis). The problem was, there was no such knowledge. Not yet. Probably not ever. But the belief that there *was* such knowledge took hold within sectors of the profession, which saw it as an unacceptable mode of social control. These activists subscribed to a redefining mode of their own, which they considered altruistic: mental patients were said to have been "labeled," and were *not* to be drugged. So, as the federal government turned to other matters, the mental institutions continued to release patients, essentially to fend for themselves. There was no connection made: we're quite capable of that in the public sphere.

Professor Fred Siegel of Cooper Union observed: "in the great wave of moral deregulation that began in the mid-1960's, the poor and the insane were freed from the fetters of middle-class mores" (Siegel 1992). Soon, the homeless appeared, only to be defined as victims of an insufficient supply of affordable housing. No argument, no amount of evidence has yet affected that fixed ideological view.

I mention this because science goes forward even as politics, often as not, regresses. Ours surely is the great age of discovery in the field of neuroscience. We are exploring the brain, not least with respect to the effect of drugs. Since the desire of man to alter his state of consciousness is as old as human history, and technology continues to provide a breath-taking array of drugs capable of producing everything from oblivion to nirvana, I think it safe to assume that we may never win a "war" against drugs. Perhaps the closest we can come, through scientific research, will be to identify "pre-exposure" vulnerability in the population and develop some sort of active or passive immunization.

We're making progress. So much so that in 1997 a significant portion of an issue of *Science*, the journal of the American Association for the Advancement of Science, was devoted exclusively to "The Science of Substance Abuse." It is near to vibrant in its engagement. We are getting toward science. Supply interdiction doesn't much work, although, absent it, things could be even worse. But we spend twice as much on interdiction as we do on bio-medical research. And the latter *moves*.

I was especially struck recently by the article "Addiction Is a Brain Disease, and It Matters" by Alan I. Leshner, Director of the National Institute on Drug Abuse. (The institute, incidentally, was established in 1973—one aspect of the Nixon initiative.) Leshner concludes as I would conclude:

> Addiction as a chronic, relapsing disease of the brain is a totally new concept for much of the general public, for many policymakers, and, sadly, for many health care professionals. . . .
>
> At the policy level, understanding the importance of drug use and addiction for both the health of individuals and the health of the public affects many of our overall public health strategies. An accurate understanding of the nature of drug abuse and addiction should also affect our criminal justice strategies. For example, if we know that criminals are drug addicted, it is no longer reasonable to simply incarcerate them. If they have a brain disease, imprisoning them without treatment is futile. If they are left untreated, their recidivism rates to both crime and drug use are frighteningly high; however, if addicted criminals are treated while in prison, both types of recidivism can be reduced dramatically. It is therefore counterproductive to not treat addicts while they are in prison. . . .
>
> At an even more general level, understanding addiction as a brain disease also affects how society approaches and deals with addicted individuals. We need to face the fact that even if the condition initially comes about because of voluntary behavior (drug use), an addict's brain is different from a non-addict's brain, and the addicted individual must be dealt with as if he or she is in a different brain state. We have learned to deal with people in different brain states for schizophrenia and Alzheimer's disease. Recall that as recently as the beginning of this century we were still putting people with schizophrenia in prisonlike asylums, whereas now we know they require medical treatments. We now need to see the addict as someone whose mind (read: brain) has been altered fundamentally by drugs. Treatment is required to deal with the altered brain function and the concomitant behavioral and social functioning components of the illness.
>
> Understanding addiction as a brain disease explains in part why historic policy strategies focusing solely on the social or criminal justice aspects of drug use and addiction have been unsuccessful. They are missing at least half of the issue. If the brain is the core of the problem, attending to the brain needs to be a core part of the solution. (Leshner 1997, 45–47)

You have to be optimistic about the problem, because now that we are nearer to describing it appropriately, we're much closer to solving it.

The outcome of narcotics prohibition over the past century has been to concentrate drug abuse and addiction principally among an urban underclass for which there is currently little public understanding or sympathy. So Congress and the public continue to fixate on supply interdiction and harsher sentences (without treatment) as the "solution" to our drug problems, and adamantly refuse to acknowledge what Dr. Leshner and others now *know* and are telling us: that addiction is a chronic, relapsing disease; that is, the brain undergoes molecular, cellular, and physiological changes that may not be reversible.

If we acknowledge that genetics and environmental factors probably cause a portion of the population to be vulnerable to drug experimentation, abuse, and addiction, our drug control policies must necessarily change. But for the moment, while the science of drug abuse and addiction holds great therapeutic promise, the politics are self-defeating, punitive, and vainglorious.

NOTES

1. Bayer advertised heroin as "The Sedative for Coughs." After both *heroin* (1898) and *aspirin* (1899) became trademarks, Bayer announced, "We are now sending to physicians throughout the United States literature and samples of both."

2. In chapter 5 in this volume, Robert DuPont describes the heroin epidemic that struck Washington in the late 1960s and peaked in terms of first use by young African American males in 1969. This was the year in which the Nixon administration took office and was asked to garrison the capital. Dr. DuPont describes the Narcotics Treatment Administration established by the new administration and its short-lived but palpable success:

> One prominent criticism of NTA's early successes was that the program's supporters were motivated merely by a desire to reduce crime. Skeptics argued that NTA's goal was not medical, but merely political. To NTA supporters, reducing crime was obviously a medical goal. Crime has many victims, including the criminals themselves, who suffer terribly not only from imprisonment but also from the lifestyles they adopt. Reducing crime was an important public health goal; successfully reducing crime was a public health triumph. The vagaries of American political life in the 1970s did not see it that way. Crime reduction was thought to be a right-wing, mean-spirited, even racist and inhumane political goal. Besides, liberals had bigger concerns. They wanted to end poverty and racism by attacking the root causes of racism.
>
> Even conservatives, while remaining strong advocates of crime reduction, were troubled by using addiction treatment to achieve this goal. Addiction treatment was expensive, often not successful, and appeared to "coddle" addicts rather than holding them accountable for their illegal behaviors (crime and drug use). Heroin addiction treatment, especially the use of methadone, remains what it was in 1970, largely a political orphan. I wish this passage were prescribed reading in classes in the social sciences.

In 1969 I was, first, Assistant to the President for Urban Affairs and, afterward, Counselor to the President. One initiative after another—and there were many, some without precedent—was caught in the crossfire of "root causes," on the one hand, and "coddling," on the other. All hail then to James Q. Wilson and his cohorts, who have demonstrated that the most important thing to do about crime, or at least the first thing to do, is to treat the symptoms!

REFERENCES

Congressional Record 1988. 100th Cong., 2d sess. 134, no. 146 (Oct. 14).

Dole, Vincent P. 1991. Distinguished Science Lecture, Annual Meeting of the American Society of Addiction Medicine. Boston, April 19. Published as "Addiction as a Public Health Problem." *Alcoholism: Clinical and Experimental Research* 15, no. 5.

Jeckel, James F., et al. 1986. "Epidemic Free-Base Cocaine Abuse: Case Study from the Bahamas." *Lancet* 1 (1 March): 459–62.

Kelly, Raymond W., and James E. Johnson. 1998. Prepared testimony of Raymond W. Kelly, Commissioner of the U.S. Customs Service, and James E. Johnson, Undersecretary of the Treasury for Enforcement, before U.S. Senate Committee on Finance, Washington, D.C., September 3.

Kennedy, John F. 1963. In *Public Papers of President John F. Kennedy*. Washington, D.C.: U.S. Government Printing Office, 1964.

Leshner, Alan I. 1997. "Addiction Is a Brain Disease, and It Matters." *Science* 278, no. 5355 (October 3).

Moynihan, Daniel P. 1969a. Memorandum to John N. Mitchell, Attorney General, February 11. National Archives.

———. 1969b. "The Whiskey Culture and the Drug Culture." Address to Governors' Conference luncheon, U.S. Department of State, Washington, D.C., December 3. Library of Congress.

———. 1973. "Peace." Alfred E. Stearns Lecture, Andover Academy, Andover Mass., January. Published as "Peace: Some Thoughts on the 1960's and 1970's." *Public Interest* (Summer 1973).

———. 1992. "Iatrogenic Government: Social Policy and Drug Research." Norman E. Zinberg Lecture, John F. Kennedy School of Government, Harvard University, Cambridge, Mass., December 7. Published in *American Scholar* 63 (Summer 1993).

Moynihan, Daniel P., and Sam Nunn. 1988. "Epidemic: A Concept Paper by the Democratic Substance Abuse Working Group," U.S. Senate, Washington, D.C., June 29.

Musto, David F. 1973. *The American Disease*. New Haven, Conn.: Yale University Press. 3d ed., New York: Oxford University Press, 1999.

———. 1975. "Whatever Happened to 'Community Mental Health?'" *Public Interest* (Spring).

———. 1997. "America's Experience with Drugs." Paper presented at the conference "The Crack Decade: Research Perspectives and Lessons Learned." National Institute on Drug Abuse and the National Institute of Justice, Baltimore, November 4.

————. 1998. "This 10-Year War Can Be Won." *Washington Post*, June 14, p. C7.
National Center on Addiction and Substance Abuse at Columbia University.
     (CASA). 1997. *Behind Bars: Substance Abuse and America's Prison Population*.
     New York: CASA.
Public Law 100–690. 1988. 102 Stat. 4181 (November 18).
Siegel, Fred. 1992. "Reclaiming Our Public Space." *City Journal* 2, no. 2 (Spring).
————. 1997. *The Future Once Happened Here*. New York: Free Press.
Wilson, James Q., and George L. Kelling. 1982. "Broken Windows: The Police and
     Neighborhood Safety." *Atlantic Monthly*, March, pp. 29–38.
Zinberg, Norman E. 1984. *Drug, Set, and Setting: The Basis for Controlled Intoxicant
     Use*. New Haven, Conn.: Yale University Press.

3

Heroin Politics and Policy under President Nixon

Egil Krogh, Jr.

Stephen Kandall has remarked on the blame-hatred-anger syndrome. That was the dominant theme when President Nixon was elected: he was ready to take after pushers and traffickers and users and possessors, and lock them up and throw away the key. But, over a period of a year or two, he began to think that wasn't the whole answer.

In 1970 an intergovernmental study group was set up under Dr. Bertram Brown, who was then the head of the National Institute of Mental Health, to make recommendations about policy initiatives on drugs. Jeff Donfeld, a domestic policy aide, simultaneously had asked Dr. Jerome Jaffe, from Illinois, to put together a report based on the recommendations of a number of outside experts who were not directly on the federal payroll.

While these studies were going on, Vietnam was beginning to have a major impact on people's thoughts about the drug issue. In August 1970 I went to Vietnam to find out for myself how serious the drug problem was. The President had sent a back-channel message to General Creighton Abrams—"Give him anything he wants. I'm going to talk to him when he gets back"—so I had the opportunity to fly all over the country, unannounced.

I remember arriving in a firebase near the DMZ. I was wearing fatigues and boots, and I walked over to where a few fellows were sitting on their haunches, with their bandannas on and their peace symbols, and one of them was smoking something that probably would have to have been registered in Washington, D.C. I said to them, "Gentlemen, I'm here from the White

House to find out about the drug problem." This soldier looks up at me, and he takes a deep toke and says, "And I'm from Mars, man." I never forgot that. But I said, "No, really, I'm from the White House. What's available?" And he said, "You want pot? You want shit? Whatever you want, just go down there." I went to thirteen firebases, from the DMZ down to Bac Lu in South Vietnam, and that experience was replicated.

When I reported to the President, I said, "Mr. President, you don't have a drug problem in Vietnam; you have a condition. Problems are things we can get right on and solve. Conditions we have to ameliorate as best we can. I don't think we can solve this short of bringing everybody home."

At the end of 1970 the two committees gave their reports. The Brown group's advice basically was to do more of what we were doing, with some more money. With the Jaffe group, I was struck by the policy recommendations and by the political implications of possibly being able to get some results under way by early 1972, the beginning of the next presidential election year. Federal policymaking is driven in large part by the campaign years when you want to run on accomplishments.

Parenthetically, my personal relationship with Richard Nixon is significant in this context. For some reason or other, we got along; perhaps we had had the same value set. When it came to law enforcement, crime control, narcotics control, he would call me. Also, the fact that I had known John Erlichman for twenty years at that time—since I was eleven—and that Jeff Donfeld also was close to Erlichman, had a lot to do with their receptivity to recommendations that we would make later on. They trusted us.

Before I'd gone to Vietnam, Vice Admiral William P. Mack had told me that there were only one hundred addicts in the entire military. That summer two congressmen, Morgan Murphy and Robert Steele, also went over, and they reported back that over 15 percent of the soldiers in Vietnam were addicted to heroin—an astonishing number. So we felt that we had to set up a program that would address what was happening in Vietnam and also set up a national policy or strategy that would be able to bear fruit soon.

On June 14, 1971, we had a conference at the White House about the Vietnam problem. By that time there was no partisanship on the war to speak of. A producer at ABC News called up and said, "Are you going to discuss the Vietnam drug problem?" I said, "Yes, we are," and he said, "I'd like to come and film it." That was very unusual, to come to the White House and listen to the President and his top staff talk openly and candidly about the issue—here are the problems, what do we think we can do—and film it. They did, and they called it *Heroes and Heroin*. Then on June 17 we announced the Special Action Office for Drug Abuse Prevention (SAODAP), a new drug agency in the Office of the President, and Jerry Jaffe was presented to the country as the person who would be directing it, the first drug czar.

This new office was to be in place for three years. It was to be given un-precedented power. It would set a national strategy, put policy in place, and, more important than anything, it would have control over how the drug budgets were going to be allocated among the various federal departments. It was the first time that had ever been done. That was what was hard to sell to departments and agencies. I attribute success on it to Jerry Jaffe and to Bob DuPont, and to Paul Perito and Grasty Crews. Perito was chief counsel to Representative Claude Pepper's Select Committee on Crime. Crews had been a master legislative draftsman working for the Federal Reserve.

We went up to Capitol Hill and said, "We'd like to design a program that everyone can support. The President's not going to make any political hay, we're not going to attack anybody, we want the most intelligent people pos-sible who will willingly come to work for us." And Paul Perito said, "You've come to the right place." We recruited Perito to be chief counsel to SAODAP, and he recruited Grasty Crews, and they did the lion's share of drafting the legislation that gave SAODAP a statutory foundation.

Congress eventually passed the legislation without a dissenting vote in either the Senate or the House. During those years of heavy political con-flict, that seemed virtually impossible, and I attribute its success to the people who were involved—the congressmen and senators, like Senator Charles Percy of Illinois, Senator Jacob Javits of New York, and Senator Harold Hughes of Iowa. They, of course, had a chance to look at the results of the Vietnam program, which were far better than we had hoped. They said, "You have turned the corner." It was an example of how effective you can be in running public policy if you can depoliticize it, take the politics out, and that is especially true when you're dealing with a problem as serious and as acute as this was.

Law enforcement still had a part in antidrug operations. I ran a supply-oriented program that included fifty-nine countries. We were successful in getting the Turkish government to stop growing poppy for two or three years. But, as others have noted, if you squeeze one source, the product pops out somewhere else—Afghanistan, Southeast Asia, the Golden Triangle. I worked with the CIA in Burma, where some former Kuomintang bandit generals had moved from Yunnan province in China. They grew poppy east of the Salween River, and moved it by mule caravans down to laboratories in the Golden Triangle. My task was to try to put a permanent stop to that activity. I have some problems with the terminology that we used, but we'd always defined this business as a war, and in the international smuggling arena that's the way it was.

But that side of the equation wasn't as significant as other kinds of pro-grams. The President's style of working was what Bill Gates has described as the "drill-down" theory: don't trust the bureaucracy; go out, find out, get the truth, report back to me. He didn't want something wafted in to him with the idea that it would be responsive to his political agenda; he wanted what would work. The staff all became imbued with that idea. Jeff Donfeld wrote brilliant memoranda about different modalities being tried around the country. He invited actors from Daytop Village to put on a play for White House staff to educate us about living communities. Bob DuPont took me to methadone treatment clinics in the District of Columbia; Peter Bourne took me to a clinic in Atlanta; and I went with Jerry Jaffe to Chicago.

As I look back, I haven't had a better time in my working life than this three-or-four-year period. It was a kind of Camelot in policymaking, program development, budgeting, good faith, people who worked hard and liked each other. There was a major shift to emphasis on treatment coming from an administration that at the outset had not been particularly interested in drug policy.

4

One Bite of the Apple: Establishing the Special Action Office for Drug Abuse Prevention

Jerome H. Jaffe

Drug addiction and crime were high priority issues for the Nixon administration, and, for their first year and a half, they gave strong emphasis to the law enforcement aspects of these related problems. By mid-1970, however, two members of the White House Domestic Council staff, Egil (Bud) Krogh, Jr., and Jeffrey Donfeld, began to believe that street crime could be reduced by expanding the availability of treatment for heroin addicts. Krogh and Donfeld were influenced by what they had learned about the treatment program initiated by Dr. Robert DuPont in Washington, D.C., and by DuPont's belief that a decrease in crime in the District was directly related to a rapid expansion of treatment for addicts. In the summer of 1970, at Dr. DuPont's suggestion, Donfeld visited the Illinois Drug Abuse Programs, which I had established in collaboration with the University of Chicago and the state of Illinois for the treatment of heroin addicts. Donfeld became convinced that treatment could, indeed, have a positive impact.

In the fall of 1970, Donfeld asked me to recruit and chair an ad hoc committee of consultants to develop a plan for allocating new federal resources to drug abuse treatment and prevention. We submitted our recommendations to the White House in December 1970. Although the Domestic Council staff at the White House continued to work actively on the drug problem, they communicated very little to those of us who had prepared the report until the following spring. Then, in April 1971, Congressmen Morgan Murphy and Robert Steele made the startling announcement that up to 15 percent of the soldiers in Vietnam were addicted to heroin. (Nothing had been mentioned to the group of consultants that I had convened about a heroin problem in Vietnam. A later review of Donfeld's papers suggested that he, too, had been unaware of the problem.)

In May I finally heard again from members of the White House staff. This time they wanted my opinion on how the heroin problem in Vietnam might be controlled. As was the case with the ad hoc committee report, I was cautioned not to discuss the issue with anyone—a caution that precluded my obtaining anyone else's advice and consultation. I suggested that routine urine testing to detect drug use and providing treatment for anyone testing positive, *before allowing them to leave Vietnam*, would permit us to accomplish three things: to get a better estimate of the prevalence of the problem, to ensure that physically dependent servicemen would not be released into a civilian setting unequipped to provide treatment, and to give us a deterrent to heroin use.

Such routine urine testing would require a change in the Uniform Code of Military Justice, I noted, so that having a positive drug test would no longer be a basis for a court-martial or a bad conduct discharge. I was not certain that such a change in policy would be possible. Remarkably, though, in only a few weeks all of these recommendations became the basis for a Vietnam drug intervention.

Before May 1971 the White House staff had been developing plans to establish a new coordinating agency for drugs within the Department of Health, Education, and Welfare. The urgent need to deal with the heroin problem in Vietnam and the likelihood that coordination with the Veterans Administration would also be involved led to the decision to create a higher-level office within the Executive Office of the President.

On June 17, 1971, the day the program in Vietnam became operational, President Nixon announced a "war on drugs" and created the Special Action Office for Drug Abuse Prevention (SAODAP), thereby setting up a new federal structure to coordinate drug treatment and prevention efforts. The Special Action Office was also given the task of expanding drug abuse treatment throughout the country. With little notice, I was asked to be the director of the new office and was instructed publicly by President Nixon to "knock heads together" to achieve those goals. At the press conference held when the new office was announced, I stated that one of its goals would be "to make treatment so available that no addict could say he committed a crime because he couldn't get treatment." I will summarize the next two frenetic years within the following framework: the size and nature of the problem, the specific tasks and projects we undertook, the resources we had to work with, the progress made, and some lessons learned.

THE SIZE AND NATURE OF THE PROBLEM

In mid-1971 the federal government faced three very visible drug problems: heroin use appeared to be increasing, especially in urban areas, and the crime associated with it also was rising; servicemen in Vietnam were using heroin; and the use of psychedelics and marijuana by teenagers and young adults was becoming widespread. The true extent of each of these problems was unknown, but it was estimated that there were at least half a million heroin addicts nationwide. The drug-use estimating tools that are taken for granted today—the Household Survey of Drug Abuse (which periodically measures the extent of drug use), the Drug Abuse Warning Network (which measures adverse effects and deaths related to nonmedical drug use, as seen in hospital emergency rooms and medical examiners' offices), and the High School Senior Survey—did not exist. But stark evidence for the growing size of the heroin problem was easily seen in the rising numbers of heroin-related deaths reported by medical examiners' offices in several cities. There were heroin-overdose deaths among our servicemen in Vietnam, too, and there were some surveys that estimated heroin-use rates among servicemen, but it was not clear if these were estimated numbers of occasional users or of addicts.

An analysis of heroin-use trends since the early 1970s, carried out as part of the 1997 Household Survey of Drug Abuse, showed that SAODAP was created at the peak of a heroin epidemic that occurred in the late 1960s to the early 1970s (*National Household Survey* 1997). Most drug abuse experts of that time were certain that heroin addicts who were in treatment committed fewer crimes than those who were not in treatment, but very little treatment was available. For more than fifty years, the federal government and most local communities had been relying on law enforcement to deal with heroin users and traffickers. In the few states where treatment programs existed, thousands of addicts were waiting for treatment; in most states there was no treatment at all to be had. It would have been an ample burden for any new governmental organization to deal with the Vietnam and domestic treatment gaps, and to do so quickly, but, in the time-honored way of Washington, the new Special Action Office became burdened with additional goals that represented the hopes, aspirations, and concerns of a variety of interests.

As it emerged from Congress, the challenge for SAODAP went well beyond coping with the country's immediate drug problems. SAODAP was given not only the mandate to expand treatment and deal with the heroin crisis in Vietnam, but also to coordinate all the drug abuse activities of the entire federal bureaucracy so as to reduce overlap and redundancy, to develop a national strategy, and still more. The following is a short list of the tasks

SAODAP was supposed to accomplish: (1) create a new federal agency with competence to develop national policy and to evaluate and coordinate the drug-related activities of seventeen other federal agencies (which would involve persuading Congress to give SAODAP unusual powers); (2) expand treatment, especially for heroin addiction; (3) oversee and coordinate the Vietnam intervention, and design and oversee an evaluation and follow-up; (4) create the data systems by which the effectiveness of national policy could be evaluated; (5) create a science base so that research might lead to better ways to treat and prevent addiction; (6) develop a formal written national strategy for drug abuse treatment and prevention.

Each of these items is, of course, only a chapter title. Within each chapter there were a number of additional formidable tasks. For example, there were many problems to be faced if we were to expand treatment. Most of the very modest level of federal funding for treatment that did exist was provided by grants, with no obligation on the part of the recipient to deliver a specified amount of treatment at a specified quality level. Although the government could write contracts for treatment, the typical federal contract is exceedingly detailed, and a long time is required to draw up specifications and to receive and review competitive submissions.

In order to expand treatment rapidly, we needed to specify what constituted a minimum level of treatment for each person. By doing so, SAODAP probably developed the first capitated treatment system, in which the federal government offered to pay a given amount for each patient-year of treatment in a variety of programs, including therapeutic communities and methadone maintenance. We believed there was some urgency to do this. It takes a long time for money appropriated by Congress to be translated into effective treatment at the community level. As director of SAODAP, I believed that there might be only one bite at this apple of opportunity. If the new emphasis on treatment did not begin to alter some of the measures of public concern—such as waiting lists, overdose deaths, and crime—the national sentiment would quickly swing back to its traditional emphasis on law enforcement and supply control (Musto 1999; Massing 1998).

Expanding treatment capacity and developing acceptable regulations for methadone maintenance were highly visible and highly controversial activities that were also very costly in terms of political capital, but formed only one part of treatment expansion. Expansion of methadone treatment was a centerpiece of the report the ad hoc committee prepared for the White House. It was obvious to me that in selecting me to head the Special Action Office the White House had decided to accept this recommendation.

Compared with the current pace of efforts to revise federal regulations for opioid maintenance treatment, it is amazing how quickly we were able to accomplish the steps needed for the regulatory scheme. We did it in less than one year. The effort required negotiating with the Food and Drug Administration (FDA), working out confidentiality regulations, and specifying the basic elements of treatment. Here again there was a sense of urgency. We were already seeing a strong reaction against methadone maintenance, fueled in part by reports of methadone- related deaths and the shoddy practices of some doctors, who sought to profit from the demand for this type of treatment.

Most of the resistance, however, was based not on problems with methadone but with the departure from the principle of total abstinence: it was seen as "substituting one addiction for another." The methadone "regulations" that SAODAP fostered represented a unique and somewhat unprecedented approach to a controversial aspect of medical practice (Institute of Medicine 1995). We used a device that was a hybrid of a new drug application and an investigatory new drug application. This device was intended to accomplish several goals: (1) to make it clear that methadone treatment should no longer be viewed as untested research; (2) to ease the overly restrictive regulations that the FDA had put into place in early 1971; (3) to specify the minimum level of treatment that would be acceptable, so as to permit federal funding of programs and to eliminate the "script doctors" (the physicians who would write prescriptions for addicts); (4) to reduce methadone diversion; and (5) to preempt plans by the Justice Department to introduce legislation that would have given the Bureau of Narcotics and Dangerous Drugs the authority to regulate what was essentially a medical treatment. That legislation would be rationalized on the basis of the need to prevent the diversion of methadone.

It was SAODAP's intention to increase not only the number of treatment programs in the country but also their patient capacity and geographic distribution. We wanted to develop facts on the ground to establish the existence of a wide constituency for treatment, to avoid having the drug problem appear to be solely an inner-city problem, since in fact it was not. Within the first eighteen months following the creation of SAODAP, the number of communities with federally supported drug treatment programs increased from 54 to 214, and the number of programs rose to almost 400. In SAODAP's first two years of operation more federally supported treatment capacity was developed across the nation than had been developed over the previous fifty years. Despite criticism from some quarters that SAODAP emphasized only methadone treatment, the evidence shows clearly that, measured in terms of patient capacity, therapeutic communities and drug-free programs were given more support than methadone programs (Strategy Council on Drug Abuse 1973; SAODAP 1973).

In the long run, a national treatment system cannot be run primarily from Washington. For this reason, in drafting the legislation that formally established SAODAP, our office negotiated for the inclusion of a formula grant program that would fund drug-abuse treatment agencies at the state level. Developing working relationships with fifty state-level agencies was not initially a welcome addition to the list of tasks for our fledgling agency; but, as it has turned out, fifty state-level constituencies have served the field well as congressional enthusiasm for funding treatment has waxed and waned.

It was obvious from the outset of SAODAP's efforts that the infrastructure for expanding treatment, especially the availability of a skilled workforce, simply did not exist. Most medical schools, for example, did not cover addiction or its treatment. SAODAP promoted the establishment of a program of "career teachers," which provided support for at least one faculty member at each medical school to introduce the topic of alcohol and drug addiction into the preclinical and clinical curriculum. We also established a national training center for counselors.

The Vietnam intervention I designed continued to be a front-burner issue for SAODAP for almost the entire first two years of its existence. There were numerous congressional committees that required hearings and testimony. The results of the urine testing, which were summarized monthly by the Department of Defense, seemed to indicate that the testing program was having the intended deterrent effect. With each passing month, fewer military personnel were testing positive for opiates at time of departure from Vietnam. Urine specimens confirmed positive for heroin by gas chromatography fell from about 5 percent in early July 1971 to less than 2 percent by March 1972.

I used these data repeatedly to point out both to White House staff and to Congress that "sometimes less is more." While all the military police and electronic fences and threats of court-martial could not bring heroin use under control, it was being reduced by properly arranged contingencies, even though the severity of the adverse consequence for a positive drug test had been reduced from a bad conduct discharge to a brief period of detoxification. The argument I presented internally within the executive branch was that, with respect to reducing the harm associated with illicit drug use, more can be accomplished by demand reduction than by supply control. These arguments were temporarily effective, as can be seen from the budget allocations of 1971 through 1974. The bulk of the federal drug budget during that period was devoted to demand reduction activities: treatment, prevention, and research (Strategy Council on Drug Abuse 1973). For a brief interval, policy was driven by data and results, and the Special Action Office was showing that at least one of its programs—the intervention in the military—was effective.

Immediately after I returned from inspecting the drug testing and detoxification programs in Vietnam in July 1971, I made arrangements for Dr. Lee Robins, of Washington University in St. Louis, to conduct a follow-up study to find out what happened to the servicemen who had used heroin during their tour of duty. Dr. Robins began the study in September 1971, selecting a sample of men who had left Vietnam that month. She presented the results of the one-year follow-up to SAODAP in 1973. The findings of that study were remarkable in the light of what we believed about heroin addiction up to that time. First, 42 percent of Army enlisted men had tried heroin, and about half of those who had tried it (about 20 percent) had become heroin-dependent—that is, they experienced withdrawal symptoms when they tried to stop (Robins 1973). Given that only 5 percent of the men had had confirmed heroin-positive urine tests during the very early months of the testing program, the addiction rate was somewhat higher than I had expected. One possible explanation was that some of the servicemen who had used heroin prior to September 1971 were able to stop in order to avoid detection.

Another factor that must also be considered in reconciling the results of urine tests and the findings of the study by Dr. Robins is that the urine-testing program in Vietnam initially (and for several months thereafter) involved all service personnel, from high-ranking officers to the lowest-level enlisted personnel, and covered all services—Army, Navy, and Air Force. It quickly became apparent that heroin use was hardly ever seen in officers above the rank of sergeant and that use was substantially lower in the Navy and Air Force than among Army enlisted personnel (a term that in this situation includes draftees). The purpose of focusing on Army enlisted men in the follow-up study was to increase the likelihood of finding men who had used heroin while in Vietnam. Because of these differences in sampling, the higher use rates found in the follow-up study are not necessarily inconsistent with the results from the urine-testing program.

While the high rates of heroin dependence among Army enlisted personnel were unexpected, what was even more unexpected was a relapse rate one year later of only 5 percent. In other words, 95 percent of the men who were found to be heroin-dependent while in Vietnam had not become readdicted to heroin after returning home, although some had access to opiates and actually had used them. Only a small fraction had received any treatment for addiction, although some had gone through detoxification in Vietnam. (Robins 1973, 1974, 1993). When these findings were made public, some people asserted that the results had been "spun" by the Nixon administration to make the urine-testing intervention seem more effective. Dr. Robins gave critics the opportunity to look at the data, however, and gradually they were accepted (Robin 1993). The Vietnam follow-up study, which could not have been carried out without the full support of the White House, is now recognized as a landmark in understanding the natural history of heroin addiction.

ESTABLISHING RESEARCH AS THE FOUNDATION
FOR RATIONAL POLICY

It was obvious to me long before I headed SAODAP that more resources were needed for research on drug abuse. Such an increase in research funding was recommended in the report that the ad hoc advisers submitted to the White House in December 1970. It is useful to be reminded how little research support there was at the time. The total amount of money allocated to all federal demand-side activities and law enforcement efforts having to do with drug abuse by the last Johnson administration budget in 1969 was less than $100 million (Musto 1999; Strategy Council on Drug Abuse 1973). About half of that amount was devoted to prevention and treatment, including the costs of operating the civil commitment programs at Lexington and Fort Worth. Although the prevention and treatment budget increased in 1970, the total amount allocated in the initial fiscal year (FY) 1971 budget to all basic, clinical, epidemiological, and evaluation research for all federal agencies was about $12 million, and much of this turned out to be devoted to psychopharmacological research only remotely related to problems of drug abuse. The 1971 supplementary amendment doubled the research budget, which was further expanded over the next three fiscal years.

One of SAODAP's important policy decisions, not often mentioned, concerned what it refused to do. At the time the office was created, the bulk of federal resources for treatment went to support the 1966 Narcotic Addict Rehabilitation Act, which included civil commitment as an alternative to prison and "voluntary" civil commitment for addicts not under criminal charges. Despite considerable pressure from some members of Congress to do so, SAODAP refused to expand support for involuntary treatment until there was adequate capacity to meet the needs of addicts clamoring for treatment. There was, in fact, an unpublished report available to federal agencies which argued that the civil commitment system was not working very well and that those addicts rejected as not being suitable for treatment had done almost as well at follow-up as those who received some inpatient treatment at Lexington and were subsequently seen as outpatients in the community (Mandell and Ansell 1973).

Recognizing the importance of linking treatment and the criminal justice system, SAODAP, in collaboration with the Law Enforcement Assistance Administration of the Department of Justice, designed and launched a nationwide program called Treatment Alternatives to Street Crime (TASC). Under this program, a drug user who came before the courts could enter a treatment program instead of going to jail, and progress in treatment would be considered by the courts in making final disposition on the offenses with which the addict was charged. The TASC programs, many of which were made permanent with state and local support, provided the conceptual basis for the now- popular drug courts.

A long list can be made of initiatives and actions taken by SAODAP in its first two years of existence, many of which are still in place (Jaffe 1994). Not the least of these are the federal confidentiality regulations that allow patients seeking treatment for drug use to feel confident that this informa- tion will not be disclosed and, particularly important, that it cannot be ob- tained by law enforcement agencies seeking evidence against them. The Veterans Administration multisite study of the synthetic opioid l-acetyl- methadol, which was funded entirely by SAODAP, provided one of the pivotal studies that permitted the approval of that drug by the FDA, albeit almost twenty years after the study was completed. Similarly, the study of naltrexone funded by SAODAP was important in its later approval.

RESOURCES

The federal drug budget published in the National Strategy for 1998 was about $16 billion. By that standard, the economic resources that could be influenced by SAODAP were quite small: the entire budget for treatment, prevention, and research was only $239 million in 1972 (Jaffe 1994). How- ever, the baseline funding had been so low that the new resources we were able to bring to bear on the problem represented a manyfold increase or even, in some cases, the very first resources available. Further, the growth of fed- eral funding for research, treatment, and training took place over the next two years and then flattened out, with the balance between support for sup- ply control and demand reduction activities from 1972 through 1974 shift- ing in the direction of demand reduction. By 1974 the total budget for the drug problem had reached a little over $750 million. Two-thirds of this fund- ing was devoted to treatment, research, education, and prevention. Accord- ing to an analysis by the Institute of Medicine, when adjusted for inflation, the absolute level of support for treatment and prevention was actually lower in 1989 than it was in 1974 (Institute of Medicine 1990). Though the 1974 proportion of resources allocated to demand-side activities has not been main- tained over the years, SAODAP's early decisions provided a solid beginning for research and a foundation for later expansion.

The most important resource SAODAP had was the President's backing. Although I did not have Cabinet status as director of the new office, I had been launched on my new job with his very public and graphic instruction to make sure things got done, and no one doubted President Richard Nixon's toughness in dealing with the apparatus of government. After extended ne- gotiations with Congress, SAODAP was given a power that, to the best of my knowledge, several subsequent offices with similar missions have not had:

the authority, within limits, to move money from one agency to another—
an authority usually reserved solely to the President and the Office of
Management and Budget.

Staffing the new office in 1971 was a blessing and a curse. The size of the
pool of knowledgeable and talented people in the field, in or out of government, was far, far smaller than it is today. Furthermore, very few involved with
treatment of addiction wanted to have anything to do with the Nixon administration, and the great majority were sufficiently outspoken opponents
to preclude them as potential recruits, at least initially. Much to my surprise,
the White House staff gave me virtually free rein to select people based solely
on competence and expertise. The people whom SAODAP recruited were
the hardest-working and most competent group of people I have ever had
the privilege of working with. As the years have passed, I have come to appreciate what an extraordinary time that was and what a supremely competent and dedicated group of colleagues I had at the Special Action Office.

ACHIEVEMENTS, LESSONS, AND LEGACIES

Perhaps the most lasting accomplishment of SAODAP was to restore some
balance to the national response to illicit drug use, after fifty years of emphasis
on controlling the supply of illicit drugs, and arresting and imprisoning those
caught possessing even small amounts. We developed an infrastructure for
treatment that is largely still in place—an infrastructure that recognized the
heterogeneity of the drug-using population and the need for several different types of treatment. While we are generally credited, or in some cases
blamed, for establishing methadone as a legitimate form of treatment, this
was only one of a number of steps we took to build the treatment system.

SAODAP also introduced and implemented the notion that a coherent
and rational national strategy should specify its goals and assumptions, and
put into place the mechanisms to measure whether its strategies are working. We put into place a number of the measurements that are still used to
assess the effectiveness of policy: the repeated Household Surveys, the DAWN
system, and measurements of treatment capacity. The resources and policies
for an invigorated research effort were put into place over the three budget-
ary cycles that preceded the creation of the National Institute on Drug Abuse
(NIDA). Federal support for research on the efficacy of treatment obviously
flowed from the decision to support treatment with federal funds. SAODAP
had emphasized the importance of research even before NIDA came into
being. The Vietnam follow-up and the Veterans Administration study of
1-acetylmethadol are only two of a much larger number of initiatives that
represent lasting legacies. The results of the Vietnam study shed new light
on the nature of heroin addiction, the role of treatment, and the absolute

need for using appropriate controls in research on treatment (Robins 1993). All of the research supported one of the major policy assumptions of the Special Action Office: that addicts are a heterogeneous population who need to be offered a range of treatment interventions.

Perhaps the major achievement of the Special Action Office for Drug Abuse Prevention was that treatment of addiction—and research, as well as prevention—became accepted as integral parts of the national strategy. In the FY 1974 budget, the last one that I submitted, two-thirds of the $784 million devoted to drug-abuse and drug-traffic prevention was targeted at treatment, education, and research. For one brief period in the history of drug policy, investment in demand reduction was given priority over supply control and law enforcement.

REFERENCES

Institute of Medicine. 1990. *Treating Drug Problems*, vol. 1. Edited by D. R. Gerstein and H. J. Harwood. Washington, D.C.: National Academy Press.

———. 1995. *Federal Regulation of Methadone Treatment*. Edited by R. A. Rettig and A. Yarmolinsky, Washington, D.C.: National Academy Press.

Jaffe, J. H. 1994. "Science, Policy, Happenstance: The Nathan B. Eddy Lecture." *NIDA Research Monograph* 152:18–32.

Mandell, W., and Z. Ansel. 1973. "Status of Addicts Treated Under the NARA Program." Unpublished report. Baltimore: Office of Wallace Mandell, Johns Hopkins University.

Massing, M. 1998. *The Fix*. New York: Simon and Schuster.

Musto, D. F. 1999. *The American Disease: Origins of Narcotic Control*. 3d ed. New York: Oxford University Press.

National Household Survey on Drug Abuse. Preliminary Results, 1997. 1997. Rockville, Md.: Department of Health and Human Services, Substance Abuse and Mental Health Services Administration.

Robins, L. N. 1973. *A Follow-up of Vietnam Drug Users*. Special Action Office Monograph Series A, no. 1. Washington, D. C.: U.S. Government Printing Office.

———. 1974. *The Vietnam Drug User Returns*. Special Action Office Monograph Series A, no. 2. Washington, D.C.: U.S. Government Printing Office.

———. 1993. "Vietnam Veterans' Rapid Recovery from Heroin Addiction: A Fluke or Normal Expectation?" *Addiction* 88: 1041–54.

Special Action Office for Drug Abuse Prevention (SAODAP). 1973. *First Annual Report*. Washington, D.C.: U.S. Government Printing Office.

Strategy Council on Drug Abuse. 1973. *Federal Strategy for Drug Abuse and Drug Traffic Prevention*. Washington, D.C.: The Strategy Council.

5

Is Drug Addiction a Brain Disease?

Sally Satel

More than 100 substance-abuse experts gathered in Chantilly, Virginia, in November 1995, for a meeting called by the government's top research agency on drug abuse. A major topic was whether the agency, the National Institute on Drug Abuse (NIDA), which is part of the National Institutes of Health, should declare drug addiction a disease of the brain. The experts—academics, public health workers, state officials, and others—said yes, overwhelmingly.

At the time the answer was controversial, but since then, the notion of addiction as a brain disease has become widespread, thanks in large measure to a full-blown public education campaign by NIDA which disseminated eye-catching pictures of addicts' brains under PET scan to show how the cocaine-damaged parts of the brain were "lit up"—an "image of desire," as one researcher called it.

Dramatic visuals are seductive and lend scientific credibility to NIDA's position, but politicians should resist this medicalized portrait for at least two reasons. First, it appears to reduce a complex human activity to a slice of damaged brain tissue. Second, and more important, it vastly underplays the reality that much of addictive behavior is voluntary.

Although some of those experts who met in Chantilly would say that emphasizing the role of will, or choice, is just an excuse to criminalize addiction, the experience of actually treating addicts suggests that such an orientation provides grounds for therapeutic optimism. It means that the addict is capable of self-control—a much more encouraging conclusion than one could ever draw from a brain-bound, involuntary model of addiction.

The brain-disease model leads us down a narrow clinical path. Since it implies that addicts cannot stop using drugs until their brain chemistry is back to normal, it overemphasizes the value of pharmaceutical intervention. At the same time, because the model also says that addiction is a "chronic and relapsing" condition, it diverts attention from truly promising behavioral therapies that challenges the inevitability of relapse by holding patients accountable for their choices.

WHAT DOES "BRAIN DISEASE" MEAN?

A NIDA article entitled "Addiction Is a Brain Disease, and It Matters," published in October 1997 in the prestigious journal *Science*, summarizes the evidence that long-term exposure to drugs produces addiction—that is, the compulsion to take drugs—by eliciting specific neurons in the central nervous system (Leshner 1997). Because these changes are presumed to be irreversible, the addict is perpetually at risk for relapse.

Thus, "addiction as a brain disease" means that compulsive drug-taking is driven by drug-induced brain changes. This assumes a correlation between drug-taking behavior and PET scan appearance, though such a correlation has yet to be clearly demonstrated, and it is speculated, on the basis of preliminary evidence, that subtle changes persist for years. The assumption seems to be that the neuroscience of addiction will give rise to pharmaceutical remedies. But to date, the search for a cocaine medication has come up empty. Moreover, the disposition to use drugs commonly persists among heroin addicts even after they have been treated with the best medication for normalizing the compulsion for heroin—methadone. That is because methadone does not, cannot, quell the underlying anguish for which drugs like heroin and cocaine are the desperate remedy.

A *Time* magazine article entitled "Addiction: How We Get Hooked" (Nash 1997) asked, "Why do some people fall so easily into the thrall of alcohol, cocaine, nicotine, and other addictive substances. . . ? (p. 69)" The answer, it said, "may be simpler than anyone dared imagine": dopamine, "the master molecule of addiction. . . . As scientists learn more about how dopamine works, the evidence suggests that we may be fighting the wrong battle [in the war on drugs]" (pp. 69–70). Among the persons quoted is Nora Volkow, a PET expert at Brookhaven Laboratories, who says, "Addiction . . . is a disorder of the brain no different from other forms of mental illness" (p. 70). The new insight, *Time* intones, may be the "most important contribution" of the dopamine hypothesis to the fight against drugs (p. 70).

Given the exclusive biological slant and naïve enthusiasm of the *Time* article, one is not surprised at its omission of an established fact of enormous clinical relevance: that the course of addictive behavior can be influenced by the very consequences of the drug-taking itself. When the addict reacts to adverse consequences of drug use—economic, health, legal, and personal— by eventually quitting drugs, reducing use, changing his pattern of use, or getting help, he does so voluntarily. Rather than being the inevitable, involuntary product of a diseased brain, these actions represent the essence of voluntariness. The addict's behavior can be modified by knowledge of the consequences. Involuntary behavior cannot.

INTERRUPTING THE ADDICTIVE PROCESS

In reality, the compulsion to take drugs does not dominate an addict's minute-to-minute or day-to-day existence. There are times when he is capable of reflection and purposeful behavior. During a cocaine addict's week, there are periods when he is neither engaged in a binge nor wracked with intense craving for the drug. Similarly, during the course of a heroin addict's day, he may feel calm and his thoughts may be lucid when he is confident of access to the drug and is using it in doses adequate to prevent withdrawal symptoms but not large enough to be sedating. At these times, the addict is not the helpless victim of a brain disease.

Society can legitimately place expectations and demands on addicts because their "brain disease" is not a persistent state. By contrast, it would be unthinkable to expect "victims" of true involuntary disease to control their afflictions. We would never demand that an epileptic marshal her will power to control a seizure, or that a breast cancer patient stop her tumor from metastasizing. Experimental evidence shows, however, that addicts can control drug-taking. In his book *Heavy Drinking: The Myth of Alcoholism as a Disease* (Fingarette 1989, chap. 2), philosopher Herbert Fingarette refutes the premise that alcoholism represents an inevitable total loss of control. He cites numerous independent investigations conducted under controlled conditions in behavioral laboratories showing the degree to which alcoholics are capable of regulating themselves. Researchers found, for example, that the amount of alcohol consumed was related to its cost and the effort required to obtain it. Once offered small payments, subjects were able to refuse freely available alcohol. And after they had drunk an initial "priming" dose, the amount they subsequently consumed was inversely proportionate to the size of the payment.

Fingarette acknowledges that these results were obtained with hospitalized alcoholics who were also receiving social support and help. Other experiments showed that the drinkers' beliefs and attitudes about alcohol influenced how much they consumed.

The story of the returning Vietnam servicemen is a revealing natural experiment that "changed our views of heroin," according to epidemiologist Lee Robins and colleagues, who wrote the now classic paper on the subject (Robins et al. 1980). They found that only 14 percent of men who were dependent on heroin in Vietnam—and who failed a publicized urine test at departure—resumed regular heroin use within three years of their return home. The rest had access to heroin and initially some of them even used it occasionally. What made them decide to stop for good, Robins found, was the "sordid" culture surrounding heroin use, the price of the drug (the demand for heroin and cocaine is price-elastic), and fear of arrest.

"CHRONIC AND RELAPSING" BRAIN DISEASE?

Given the heavy biomedical orientation at NIH, a signature like "chronic brain disease" is a device that aligns NIDA's mission with its parent's. Away from home, the major political purpose of the model is to establish a moral and clinical equivalence between addiction and other medical conditions. Diabetes, asthma, and high blood pressure are the trio most often cited as prototypical "chronic and relapsing" disorders. NIDA predicts that medicalization will destigmatize compulsive drug-taking and shift the commonly held perception of addicts from "bad people" to be dealt with by the criminal justice system to "chronic illness sufferers" to be triaged to medical care. In the words of a recent NIDA report, "Vigorous and effective leadership is needed to inform the public that addiction is a medical disorder. . . . [It is not] self-induced or a failure of will" (NIDA 1997: 9).

This is also the agenda of the newly formed group Physician Leadership on National Drug Policy, whose prestigious members include the former president of the AMA, a Nobel Prize winner, leaders at the Department of Health and Human Services, a former FDA director, and a former surgeon general. Eliminating stigma is also important to the Institute of Medicine. "Addiction . . . is not well understood by the public and policymakers. Overcoming problems of stigma and misunderstanding will require educating the public . . . about the progress made," a 1997 report says (Institute of Medicine 1997; see also JAMA 278, no. 5 (1997): 378).

By changing popular opinion, these institutions hope to work through federal and state legislatures to secure more treatment, expanded insurance coverage, and other services for addicts as well as more funding for addiction research. These are not unreasonable aims insofar as substandard quality of care, limited access to care, and understudied research questions remain active problems. But the destigmatizing approach has been too readily borrowed from the mental health community. Along with the obvious deterrent value, stigmatizing is necessary to help enforce societal norms. Furthermore, forcing a rigid barrier between the so-called medical and moral arenas eclipses one of the most promising venues for anti-addiction efforts: the criminal justice system (the courts and probation services), which can impose sanctions that greatly deter relapse.

In their *Lancet* article "Myths about the Treatment of Addiction," researchers Charles P. O'Brien and A. Thomas McLellan argue that (1) relapse in long-term conditions like asthma, diabetes, and hypertension is often due to the patient's poor compliance with prescribed diet, exercise, or medication; (2) an addict's relapse is a result of poor compliance; and thus (3) addiction is like other diseases (O'Brien and McLellan 1996).

But this is reversed. Asthmatics and diabetics who resist their doctor's orders resemble addicts, rather than addicts' resembling them. Asthmatics and diabetics may deteriorate spontaneously for physical reasons that are unprovoked and unavoidable; by contrast, relapse to addiction invariably represents a failure to comply with "doctors' orders"—that is, to stop using drugs.

What's more, relapse is not inevitable. A large Epidemiologic Catchment Area (ECA) study conducted in 1991 found that 59 percent of roughly 1,300 respondents who met the criteria for being considered habitual users at some point in their lives were free of drug problems at the time of interview. The average duration of remission was 2.7 years, and the mean duration of illness was 6.1 years, with about three-fourths of the cases lasting no more than eight years (Anthony and Helzer 1991). Because the ECA, which surveyed a total of 20,300 adults, did not analyze drug abuse and drug dependence separately, it is impossible to know how the two differed: presumably, dependent users had longer durations of active symptoms and shorter remissions. Even so, these figures suggest that addiction is not an enduring problem in everyone it afflicts.

DRUG CURES FOR DRUG ADDICTION?

The pharmacological imperative is a logical outgrowth of placing the brain at the center of the addictive process. Still, attempts to treat addiction with other drugs or medications have been around for centuries. In the NIDA budget, about 15 percent goes to the Medications Development Division (MDD), which was authorized by Congress in 1992. One of NIDA's major goals was the development of an anti-cocaine medication by the turn of the twenty-first century. But no magic bullet is streaking across the horizon, and the NIDA director has downgraded predictions about the curative power of medication, promoting it as potentially "complementary" to behavioral therapy.

It is always possible, of course, that an effective drug will be developed. For the sake of the public's trust and NIDA's credibility, it is important, however, that the brain-disease advocates not oversell the promise of medications. To date, more than forty pharmaceuticals have been studied in randomized controlled trials in human beings for their effect on cocaine abuse or dependence. Some of these were intended to block craving, others to substitute for cocaine itself; none has yet proved even minimally effective. The basic problem with the anti-craving medications is their lack of specificity. Instead of deploying a surgical strike on the neuronal site of cocaine yearning, they end up blunting motivation in general and may also depress mood. Experiments with substitution drugs (e.g., cocaine-like substances such as methylphenidate) have proven equally frustrating because, instead of suppressing the urge to use, they tend to act like an appetizer, producing physical sensations and emotional memories reminiscent of cocaine itself and consequently triggering a desire for the real thing.

If a selective medication could be developed, it might be especially helpful to cocaine addicts who have been abstinent for a time but who experience a sudden burst of craving for the drug, a feeling that is often reported as alien, coming from "out of nowhere," and different from a true desire to use cocaine. Such a craving may be triggered by some kind of environmental cue, such as passing through the neighborhood where the addict used to get high. Generally, the recovering addict learns his idiosyncratic cues, avoids them, and arms himself with exercises and strategies (e.g., immediately calling a twelve-step sponsor) that help him fight the urge. It is conceivable that a medication could help suppress the jolt of desire and, ultimately, derail the cue from the conditioned response.

Another approach to addiction is behavioral "extinction," a process exploited by an available anti-heroin medication called naltrexone. Naltrexone blocks opiate molecules at the site of attachment to receptors on the neuron. Both naltrexone and the cocaine vaccine create a situation in which an addict who takes the illicit drug will feel little or no effect. Uncoupling the desired response (getting high) from the action intended to produce it (shooting up) is called "extinction," and according to behaviorist theory, the addict will eventually stop using a drug if he no longer achieves an effect. Although naltrexone is technically effective, most heroin addicts reject it in favor of methadone, which can give a mild high and has a calming effect. There are a few groups, however, who will take naltrexone with good results: impaired professionals (e.g., doctors, lawyers, nurses) who risk loss of their license, and probationers and defendants on work release who are closely supervised and urine-tested frequently.

Optimism surrounding the pharmaceutical approach to drug dependence stems from the qualified success of methadone, an opiate painkiller that was developed by German chemists during World War II. First tested in 1964 as a substitute for heroin in the United States, methadone is now administered in maintenance clinics to about 19 percent of the nation's estimated 600,000 heroin addicts. Numerous studies have documented the socioeconomic benefits of methadone: significant reductions in crime, overdoses, unemployment, and, in some regions, HIV.

Unlike heroin, which needs to be administered every four to eight hours to prevent withdrawal symptoms, methadone requires a single daily dose. As a combination substitute and blocker, methadone subdues the craving for heroin. In addiction, an addict on methadone maintenance who takes heroin will be blocked from experiencing a potent high. Like the drug for which it substitutes, methadone is addictive.

Despite methadone's virtue as a substitution therapy, as many as 35 to 60 percent of those taking it also use cocaine or other illicit drugs or black-market sedatives. A six-year followup of treated addicts found that over half were readmitted to their agency at some point. This is not surprising. Methadone will only prevent withdrawal symptoms and the related physiological hunger for heroin. To be sure, a heroin addict who is given this opiate is much more likely to stay engaged in a treatment program, but methadone cannot make up for the psychic deficits that led to addiction, such as deep-seated intolerance of boredom, depression, stress, anger, and loneliness. The addict who began heavy drug use in his teens has not even completed the maturational tasks of adolescence; he has not developed social competence, consolidated a personal identity, or formed a concept of his future. Furthermore, methadone cannot solve the secondary layer of troubles that accumulate over years of drug use: family and relationship problems, educational deficiencies, health problems, economic losses. Consequently, only a small fraction of heroin addicts are able to become fully productive on methadone alone.

The failure to recognize this clinical reality was evident at a NIH-NIDA conference called "The Medical Treatment of Heroin Addiction" held in November 1997. So pervasive was the idea that a dysfunctional brain is the root of addiction that not once during the entire two-and-a-half-day meeting did any of the attendees hear such words as "responsibility," "choice," or "character"—the vocabulary of personhood. In fairness, speakers did acknowledge the importance of so-called psychosocial services, but they tended to view these as add-ons, helpful offerings to "keep" patients in the clinic while methadone, the core treatment, did its job (see NIDA 1997).

CONCLUDING OBSERVATIONS

Labeling addiction a chronic and relapsing brain disease succeeds more as sloganism than as public health education. By locating addiction in the brain, not the person, NIDA has generated an unwarranted level of enthusiasm about pharmacology for drug addiction.

The fact that many, perhaps most, addicts are in control of their actions and appetites for circumscribed periods of time shows that they are not perpetually helpless victims of a chronic disease. They are instigators of their addiction, just as they are agents of their own recovery—or nonrecovery. The potential for self-control should allow society to endorse the expectations and demands of addicts that would never be made of someone with a true involuntary illness. Making such demands is, of course, no assurance that they'll be met. But confidence in their very legitimacy would encourage a range of policy and therapeutic options—using consequences and coercion—that is incompatible with the idea of a no-fault brain disease.

Efforts to neutralize the stigma of addiction by convincing the public that the addict has a "brain disease" are understandable, but in the long run they have no more likelihood of success than the use of feel-good slogans to help a child acquire "self-esteem." Neither respectability nor a sense of self-worth can be bestowed; both must be earned. The best way for any institution, politician, or advocate to combat the stigma of addiction is to promote conditions—both within treatment settings and in society at large—that help the addict develop self-discipline and, along with it, self-respect. In this way, former addicts become visible symbols of hard work, responsibility, and lawfulness—all of which are potent antidotes to stigma.

This prescription does not deny whatever biological or psychological vulnerabilities individuals might have. Instead, it makes their struggle to master themselves all the more ennobling.

REFERENCES

Anthony, James C., and John E. Helzer. 1991. "Syndromes of Drug Abuse and Dependence." In *Psychiatric Disorders in America: The Epidemiologic Area Catchment Study*. Edited by L. N. Robins and D. A. Regier. New York: Free Press, Chap. 6.

Fingarette, Herbert. 1989. *Heavy Drinking: The Myth of Alcoholism as a Disease*. Berkeley: University of California Press.

Institute of Medicine. 1997. "Physician Leadership in National Drug Policy." Consensus Statement. July 9.

JAMA 278, no. 5 (1997). Medical News and Perspectives section.

Leshner, Alan I. 1997. "Addiction Is a Brain Disease, and It Matters." *Science* 278, no. 5355 (October 3).

Nash, J. Madeleine. 1997. "Addiction: How We Get Hooked." *Time* (May 9), 69–76.

NIDA [National Institute on Drug Abuse]. 1997. "Effective Medical Treatment of Heroin Addiction." Consensus Development Statement. Revised Draft. November 19.

O'Brien, C. P., and A. T. McLellan. 1996. "Myths about the Treatment of Addiction." *Lancet* 347: 237–40.

Robins, L. N., et al. 1980. "Vietnam Veterans Three Years after Vietnam: How Our Study Changed Our Views of Heroin." In *Yearbook of Substance Use and Abuse*, vol. 2. Edited by L. Britt and C. Winick. New York: Human Science.

Part III

The Urban Epidemic

6

Heroin Addiction in the Nation's Capital, 1966–1973

Robert L. DuPont

The modern American heroin addiction epidemic began in the nation's capital in 1966 and reached its peak in 1971. While heroin use declined dramatically in late 1972 and 1973, over the next three decades it evolved into a substantial part of a more chronic drug problem.

Between 1969 and 1973 a focused response to heroin addiction in the District of Columbia produced positive results, including fewer heroin overdose deaths and declining rates of new heroin use. The monthly rate of serious crimes in Washington, D.C., dropped by half between 1969 and 1973. While this counterpunch to the heroin epidemic was accomplished rapidly and inexpensively, most of the gains were quickly lost.

In the District of Columbia a pilot heroin addiction treatment program using methadone for outpatients was begun in the Department of Corrections in September 1969. It was expanded into the Narcotics Treatment Administration (NTA), a large multimodality addiction treatment program for the entire city within the Department of Human Resources, on February 18, 1970. While methadone remained the dominant form of care, NTA also included therapeutic communities, inpatient detoxification, and outpatient drug-free treatment.

The early success of NTA led Richard Nixon, a president with a reputation for being tough on drugs and crime, to establish a new drug policy. Although the federal government had for fifty years responded to drug addiction with a nearly total reliance on law enforcement, in 1971 Nixon created the first White House drug office and committed the federal government to unprecedented investments in addiction treatment and research. The President appointed Jerome H. Jaffe, one of the most talented leaders of the emerging addiction field, as the first White House drug czar.

NTA's major legacy was this policy shift away from an exclusive reliance on law enforcement and toward a balanced strategy that included treatment and research. The historical and political context of NTA is described in a number of publications about drug addiction (Baum 1996; Courtwright 1982; Jonnes 1996; Massing 1998b; Musto 1999). NTA was described more completely in papers presented at the Fifth National Conference on Methadone Treatment held March 17–19, 1973, in Washington, D.C. For an exploration of the problems of addiction, including treatment, prevention, and research, see *The Selfish Brain: Learning from Addiction* (DuPont 1997).

During the 1970s the NTA approach was extended to a national attack on drug addiction. For these new strategies to be accepted, many old, well-established barriers had to fall. Policymakers on both ends of the political spectrum doubted the potential for addiction treatment. Conservatives advocated a pure get-tough law enforcement approach to curb the heroin epidemic. Liberals argued that since heroin addicts were victims of racism and poverty, until those more fundamental social problems were overcome, it was futile to attack the heroin addiction epidemic.

More than political resistance hampered the ambitious use of addiction treatment to curb the heroin epidemic. After fifty years of dealing with opiate addiction, the best thinkers in American medicine believed addiction treatment did not work. High recidivism appeared to doom all forms of therapy. In addition, many people considered heroin addiction to be part of a larger "substance-abuse" problem, in which the possible focuses of abuse range from chocolate to drugs. Tobacco and alcohol products were included as part of this one, indivisible addiction situation. Some of those seeking new strategies to rein in the heroin epidemic in the early 1970s saw legalization of the drug as an attractive alternative to either law enforcement or treatment (Alsop 1972a, 1972b).

To justify a treatment-based response, it was necessary first to accept the premise that intravenous heroin addiction is a more immediately devastating problem than other addictions, and that addiction not only reflects but also causes social problems, such as poverty and crime. Second, community leaders with limited resources had to accept that the relatively small number of heroin addicts meant that a targeted response of treatment for heroin users was a realistic goal which was more achievable than attacking less well-defined problems. Third, policy leaders had to view heroin addiction as a primary problem, not merely a derivative of some other social malady. Fourth, public officials had to be convinced by new evidence in the late 1960s that heroin addiction could be successfully treated via methadone maintenance, as well as via participation in therapeutic communities.

Two central public health questions emerged once a treatment initiative was envisioned. First, could a targeted communitywide treatment response to heroin addiction be established despite deep and widespread popular resistance, particularly to the use of methadone maintenance? Second, would a major treatment effort make a difference not only for individual addicts but also for the whole community? The NTA experience answered these two questions in the early 1970s.

THE STORY OF NTA

When examining the historical backdrop of NTA, including its relationship to the sudden crime rise in the late 1960s, it is useful to refer to the reports of two distinguished presidential commissions that gathered the best thinking available on these issues (President's Commission on Crime 1966; President's Commission on Law Enforcement 1967a, 1967b). A recent review of the 1967 national report on drugs and crime noted that despite its sophistication, the report did not identify the heroin addiction epidemic or foresee the potential for addiction treatment to curb either rates of drug use or crime (DuPont and MacKenzie 1994).

During the period covered by this chapter, NTA evolved from a small, outpatient methadone treatment program for paroled heroin addicts that began September 15, 1969, into a complex multimodality program. Twenty NTA centers included residential beds, therapeutic communities, and contracts with several nonprofit community addiction treatment programs. Most NTA patients went through a medical intake procedure that included a physical examination and laboratory tests, in addition to an evaluation by an experienced counselor. After an initial central medical intake, NTA staff referred the patient to one of the NTA treatment centers, depending on the patient's preferences, the services needed, where the patient lived or worked, and the availability of treatment capacity.

Although methadone treatment had been started by Vincent Dole and Marie Nyswander, two distinguished physicians, in 1964, its legal status remained clouded in 1969, because many drug experts in the Public Health Service and many federal narcotics agents remained skeptical about, if not openly hostile to, the use of methadone in the treatment of heroin addiction. In 1970, stimulated by White House acceptance of the initial success of NTA and other pioneering programs, the federal government approved the limited use of methadone in large-scale research programs. In 1971, with a strong push from the new Special Action Office for Drug Abuse Prevention (SAODAP) in the White House, the first federal regulations were issued permitting methadone treatment outside of a research context. The Washington drug treatment program began its use of methadone in 1969 under research guidelines. Federal regulation of methadone treatment has persisted to the present, making it unique in this regard among addiction treatments, as well as in American health care (Lowinson et al. 1997, 405–15).

NTA's treatment was divided between residential and outpatient care. Over the three years covered in this chapter, a total ranging from about 12,000 to a maximum of 14,400 patients were actively in treatment at NTA at any one time. NTA treatment fell into one of three broad types: abstinence, outpatient methadone detoxification, and methadone maintenance. Abstinence, or drug-free, treatment did not involve the use of methadone at all, while detoxification from heroin addiction included decreasing methadone doses. In methadone maintenance treatment, the patient used methadone daily for many months or even years.

About 70 percent of patients entering treatment chose abstinence or detoxification, and about 30 percent chose methadone maintenance. Because patients in methadone maintenance stayed in treatment longer than those choosing abstinence or detoxification, at any given time about 60 percent of NTA patients were in methadone maintenance, about 20 percent were in methadone detoxification, and about 20 percent were in abstinence treatment.

Abstinence treatment, a popular option, included residential care for several weeks and outpatient visits for counseling over weeks or months, as well as three therapeutic community programs. Patients chose the type of abstinence care they preferred.

The most visible and controversial form of treatment at NTA was outpatient methadone maintenance treatment. The patient typically began with a gradual dose escalation from about 10 mg of methadone a day to a maximum of about 100 mg in a once-a-day oral dose. All NTA methadone patients had counselors, and each NTA treatment center had a variety of services, including counseling and vocational assistance. A typical NTA outpatient center had about two hundred patients and a staff of about twelve, of whom about six were counselors and one a vocational specialist. Patients met with their counselors several times during the first week of treatment. Visits gradually decreased to weekly, then monthly appointments. After successful daily participation for several months, methadone maintenance patients received take-home doses of methadone. Their visits declined from six or seven each week at the start to once a week after about six months. Methadone maintenance patients stayed in treatment as long as they chose, provided that they complied with NTA program requirements, including regular attendance and continued abstinence from the use of illicit drugs, as shown by frequent urine tests. Outpatient methadone detoxification involved maximum methadone doses of 40 mg or less and, typically, stays in treatment of three weeks to six months.

Regardless of their treatment modality, all patients were checked for illegal drug use by means of regular observed urine tests. Overall, NTA patients stayed in treatment an average of about four months, but some had shorter stays and others stayed active with NTA for many years. NTA focused on three objectively measured goals: nonuse of illicit drugs (especially, but not exclusively, nonuse of heroin), freedom from arrest, and employment.

One of NTA's most important innovations was the concept of a "reportable patient." To be counted as an active patient, a heroin addict needed to have shown up for at least two visits a week for the prior two weeks. This definition ensured that heroin addicts were truly involved with NTA before they were considered to be patients. The strict reporting requirement, along with computerized monitoring and uniform intake procedures, laid the basis for usable, reliable NTA data.

Growing from a pilot treatment program in the Department of Corrections, NTA came to include a program of universal drug testing for all Washington, D.C., criminal defendants. This program, the nation's first, began on April 1, 1970. The D.C. Superior Court's urine testing program for illicit drug use has continued without interruption from 1970 to the present. The links NTA forged between the criminal justice system and drug treatment, including a strong reliance on drug testing, led directly to the national Treatment Alternatives to Street Crime program supported by the White House Special Action Office for Drug Abuse Prevention and later to the drug court movement. The relationships between the criminal justice system and drug treatment have been reviewed, emphasizing the public health benefits of universal drug testing of convicted criminals on parole and probation (DuPont and Wish 1992).

NTA's rapid success culminated in a turning point in national drug policy similar to Nixon's opening of diplomatic relations with the previously pariah state of Communist China in 1972. Both were historically important new policy directions which appeared to be politically out of character for the conservative President. In contrast to his widely recognized initiative in China, Nixon's new direction in addiction policy has only recently gotten the attention it deserves (Gladwell 1998; Massing 1998a). Both policy shifts were dramatic breaks from the rigid (and bipartisanly promulgated) dogma of the past, in which the federal government's response to addiction was almost exclusively a law-enforcement response. They ushered in a new era of national policy that has achieved bipartisan support for more than a quarter of a century. During the years following the drug policy shift, federal support for treatment and research has grown in total dollars, but the percent of all federal money that goes to treatment and research has declined somewhat.

Nevertheless, this support remains clearly different from all that went before 1971. Support for methadone treatment has been less visible, but the total number of patients in methadone treatment in the country has been about level during the period, at around one hundred thousand.

PROFILE OF THE NTA PATIENT POPULATION

In October 1970, NTA computerized all of its patient records. By that time about two thousand people who had been treated in the first eight months of the program had left the NTA system. In 1973 NTA had computerized records on thirteen thousand heroin-addicted patients. Beginning with an annual budget of just over $1 million, by 1973 NTA had increased its resources to $7.5 million yearly. The agency spent about $17 million in appropriated and grant-backed funds to treat fifteen thousand patients during its first three years of operation.

Prevalence and Incidence of Use

Prevalence of heroin use is the number of people (or the percentage of a population group) who have used heroin during a specified period of time, typically one year. Incidence of heroin use is the number (or the percentage of a population group) who first used heroin during a particular period of time, also typically one year (DuPont and Greene 1973, 716–22).

The peak year of first heroin use was 1969, named by 21 percent of NTA's patients. Eighteen percent of NTA's patients first used in 1968, and 14 percent in 1970. Thus, 53 percent of NTA's patients first used heroin in just three years. The period 1968–70 was the peak of first use (incidence) during this epidemic. Two publications describe the NTA experience (DuPont and Greene 1973, 716–22; Greene and DuPont 1974, 545–50). See figure 6.1 for age at first use and year of first use for NTA patients (DuPont 1973c).

It has been estimated that about eighteen thousand D.C. residents were addicted to heroin at some point between 1970 and 1974, for a prevalence rate of about 2,400 per 100,000 during that time. The incidence of new heroin use in 1969 was estimated to be 420 per 100,000 residents. (See table 6.1 for annual incidence of heroin use from 1960 to 1973.) The estimate of 18,000 heroin addicts corresponded to about 2.2 percent of the D.C. population.

During three years NTA treated one in fifty citizens of the District of Columbia for heroin addiction. In large sections of the city, the prevalence of NTA-treated heroin use was even greater. In some neighborhoods, during those three years, more than one-quarter of the young men aged twenty to twenty-four were treated by NTA. Among black males aged fourteen to

Figure 6.1
Age and Year of First Heroin Use, NTA Patients

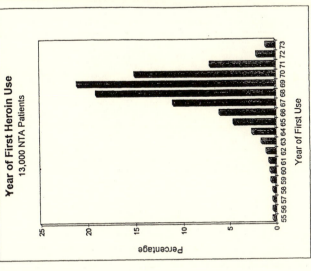

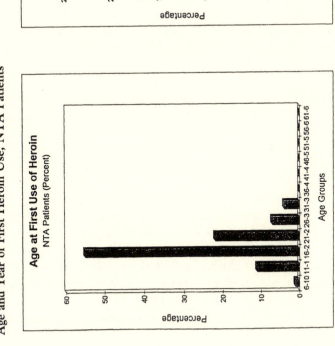

Source: Robert L. DuPont, "Perspective on an Epidemic." Washington, D.C.: Washington Center for Metropolitan Studies, 1973). Unpublished data.

Table 6.1
Annual Incidence of Heroin Use in the District of Columbia, 1960–73:
Cases per 1,000 in Three Population Groups

Year	General Population	Young Persons Age 13–25 Years	Young Black Males Age 14–25 Years
1960	0.2	0.6	1.5
1961	0.2	0.8	1.9
1962	0.3	1.0	2.5
1963	0.3	1.3	3.1
1964	0.5	2.1	5.0
1965	0.8	3.2	7.7
1966	1.2	4.8	11.6
1967	2.1	8.4	20.2
1968	3.6	14.4	34.7
1969	4.2	16.9	40.4
1970	2.9	11.9	28.5
1971	1.2	4.7	11.2
1972	0.4	1.6	3.9
1973	0.2	0.8	1.9

Source: Adapted from American Journal of Public Health Supplement 64 (December 1974): 2.

twenty-five, the incidence of new heroin use in 1969 reflected in NTA admissions was 4,040 per 1,000,000 for the population of the entire city. These data show a roughly 50 percent year-to-year rise in the incidence of heroin use for each year from 1965 to 1969.

Personal Characteristics and Admission Status of Patients

Among NTA patients, 82.1 percent were male, and 92.5 percent were black (7.4 percent were white and 0.1 percent other). Voluntary admissions represented 65.4 percent of the total, while 34.5 percent were referred to NTA from the criminal justice system (which most often was the D.C. Superior Court program). At intake 33.4 percent were employed, 62.1 percent were unemployed, and 4.4 percent were in school or training. More than half of the NTA patients (56.6 percent) were single, 23.0 percent were married, and 20.4 percent formerly had been married.

Comparison with Surrounding Community

Compared with the demographic profile of the total population of the District of Columbia in 1970, the NTA patient population was more male, more limited to young adults, and far more involved with the criminal justice system. It was somewhat more black (92.5 percent vs. 71 percent) and had about the same educational level (11.0 years vs. 11.5 years).

The average NTA patient had used heroin for four years prior to admission to NTA treatment. The most common, or *modal*, age at first heroin use was seventeen. The modal age at admission to NTA was twenty-one; average educational level was eleventh grade; average number of arrests was four, and of convictions, one. Seventy-three percent of NTA patients were between eighteen and twenty-five at intake. More than half (55 percent) of NTA's patients first used heroin between the ages of sixteen and twenty; only 5 percent first used the drug after the age of twenty-six. Eleven percent first used heroin between the ages of eleven and fifteen.

Analysis of Birth Cohorts

Focusing on birth-year cohorts derived from NTA intake forms, we examined one epidemic of initial heroin use that peaked in 1950. This epidemic was seen in birth cohorts from 1925 to 1934 (that is, people who were between the ages of sixteen and twenty-five in 1950). During this earlier epidemic, the modal age of first heroin use was eighteen, not far from the sixteen-year-old modal age for NTA patients' first use between 1970 and 1973. The sharpest peaking in the 1950 heroin epidemic occurred for NTA patients born in 1932. When the peak years of birth for each epidemic were compared, it was found that 19 percent of the 1932 birth-year cohort first used heroin in 1950, while 36 percent of the 1953 birth-year cohort first used heroin in 1969.

The larger epidemic peak of first heroin use (incidence) in 1969 was stable in birth cohorts from 1940 to 1954 (people who were age fifteen to twenty-nine in 1969), demonstrating that this peak was not a cohort effect but a stable peak of incidence of heroin use in the community as a whole. The age at the onset of heroin use was stable in a narrow range, taking place almost exclusively between fifteen and thirty, while the sharpest peak of new heroin use occurred between the ages of sixteen and twenty.

For those born in 1932, the epidemic peak of new heroin use occurred in 1950 (see figure 6.2). Birth years 1936 and 1940 do not show either of the epidemic peaks in 1950 or 1969. Addicts born in these years were initiated into heroin use primarily during endemic (or nonepidemic) years. By the birth year 1953, the 1969 epidemic of new heroin use appears (see figure 6.2). There is no other explanation for this pattern than that the District of Columbia experienced two epidemics of new heroin use: a smaller one in 1950 and a larger one in 1969.

Most patients treated by NTA were born between 1945 and 1954, the baby boom years. About 10.5 percent of males and 1.9 percent of females in this

Figure 6.2
Year of First Heroin Use for Selected NTA Male Birth Cohorts

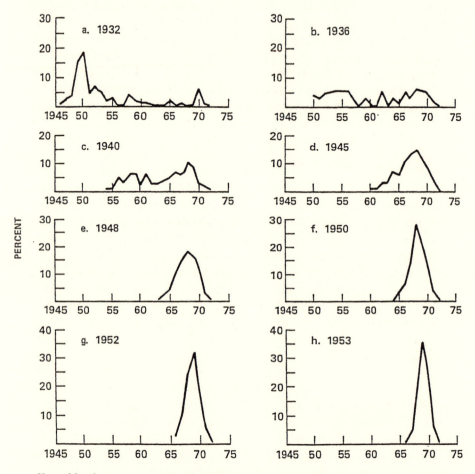

a.   Year of first heroin use among male NTA patients born in 1932. Note the peak in 1950, sug-
     gesting that Washington, D.C., like other cities in the United States, experienced a heroin
     epidemic in the post-World War II period.
b.   Typical curve for a birth cohort too young to have been affected by the 1950 epidemic and
     too old to have been affected by the epidemic in the 1960s.
c-h. Series of birth cohorts increasingly affected by the current epidemic. The peak attack rate was
     observed in males born in 1953, who were sixteen–seventeen years old in 1969.

Source: American Journal of Public Health Supplement (December 1974): 2. Reprinted by permission.
   Copyright © 1974 by the American Public Health Associations.

birth cohort in the District of Columbia in 1970 were treated for heroin addiction by 1973. Pre-epidemic attack rates of heroin addiction for adolescent males were about 0.2 percent per year, as opposed to the peak rate during the epidemic of more than 5 percent per year (DuPont 1973a). Thus the epidemic incidence was about twenty-five times the endemic incidence rate for first heroin use.

Recognizing that heroin addicts are less likely to come into treatment in the first year or two after they begin using heroin, it was possible that the sharp decline in apparent incidence of heroin use after 1969 could have been an artifact of the delay in entering treatment after initiation of heroin use. When successive six-month admission cohorts between July 1970 and July 1973 were compared, there was no shift of the year of peak incidence of first heroin use; it stayed in 1969 for all of these admission cohorts. Successive intake cohorts over this three-year period showed an increase in age at admission. In July 1970, 31 percent of NTA intakes were for people under the age of twenty-one, with half of those being under the age of eighteen. By the end of 1972, only 17 percent of patients entering treatment were under twenty-one, and only 2 percent were under eighteen; and by September 1973 only 8 percent were under twenty-one, and just 1 percent were under eighteen.

The mean age of NTA admissions rose 3.5 years in that 2.5-year period, showing not only that there was a smaller number of new heroin users in the District of Columbia over that time but also that a substantial number of younger users were then becoming nonusers of heroin, even in the absence of treatment. NTA treated over 2,500 people who first used heroin in 1969 but only 107 who first used the drug in 1973.

TRACING THE CURVE OF THE EPIDEMIC

NTA made an early decision to treat as many heroin-addicted patients who wanted care as possible. Even if this created overcrowding and stress on patients and staff, this was considered to be a sound public health decision—maximizing the benefits NTA could provide to the whole community. Between October 1971 and February 1972, approximately twenty-five new patients were admitted to NTA each business day. In March 1972 there was an increase in the demand for treatment: NTA intake soared to a peak of fifty-eight in one day. To avoid overcrowding that was severe even by NTA's standards, in April 1972 intakes of new patients were restricted to twenty-five per day. By the late summer of 1972, however, a decline in the demand for addiction treatment permitted the lifting of intake restrictions. The monthly intake peaked in March 1972 at just over one thousand. It fell during mid-1972, leveling off after September 1972 at about two hundred admissions each month. Readmissions equaled new admissions for the first time in June (for voluntary admissions) and July (for court-directed admissions) of 1972. By February 1973, readmissions were nearly twice as numerous as new admissions among both voluntary and court-directed patients. The decline in the demand for treatment at NTA facilities after March 1972 was the same for both voluntary and involuntary patients, showing that the reduced intake reflected a sharp fall in the prevalence of heroin addiction and not merely a shift in addicts' attitudes toward NTA's care. (See table 6.2 for the number of monthly NTA admissions [DuPont and Greene 1973, 716–22].)

Looking at the urine drug tests conducted at D.C. Superior Court, the rate of heroin positives peaked at 31 percent in March 1972 and fell to an all-time low for this period of 8 percent in September 1973. Four separate surveys of admissions to D.C. jails using similar techniques were conducted with the following percent positives for recent heroin use: August 1969, 30 percent; January 1971, 47 percent; August 1972, 24 percent; and February 1973, 13 percent.

Heroin overdose deaths (ODs) were first tabulated for D.C. in 1969, but death investigations became more sophisticated in 1971, when the D.C. Medical Examiner's office was created and brilliantly led by James L. Luke. Heroin overdose deaths peaked in 1971, when twenty-nine O.D.s occurred in a three-month period. The heroin overdose deaths may have fallen earlier than data show, because the new medical examiner's office was more efficient in identifying heroin-related deaths than the previous coroner system. Thus, the actual peak of heroin overdose deaths may have been 1970 rather than 1971. During 1972 there were only twenty heroin O.D.s, and the first nine months of 1973 saw only four heroin overdose deaths in Washington (Greene, Luke, and DuPont 1974, Ruttenberger and Luke 1984; see figure 6.3).

Washington's crime rate was measured by the seven FBI index crimes: robbery, burglary, larceny of more than $50, and auto theft in the property-related group; and murder, rape, and aggravated assault in the nonproperty-related offenses. As shown in figure 6.4, virtually the entire rise in D.C.'s crime rate after 1965 occurred in property-related offenses. The rate of serious crime in the District of Columbia began to decline in late 1969. If the increased police presence in 1970 and 1971 was the primary reason for the fall of serious crime, it would be expected that the property-related and the nonproperty-related crimes would have fallen in tandem, but they did not. Only changing heroin addiction rates in the District of Columbia would selectively affect the property crime rate. Similarly, only the rise in heroin use in the late 1960s can explain the selective rise in property-related crimes at that time (Kozel and DuPont 1977).

Table 6.2
Number of Monthly NTA Admissions, October 1971–February 1973

Year	Month	Voluntary Admissions		Criminal Justice Admissions		Total	Daily Average
		New	Readmit	New	Readmit		
1971	October	212	141	120	75	548	26.1
	November	250	150	197	89	686	32.7
	December	189	136	118	89	532	25.3
1972	January	175	137	104	84	500	23.8
	February	194	165	93	80	532	25.3
	March	473	325	133	99	1030	49.0
	April	306	225	88	88	707	33.7
	May	227	183	106	92	608	30.0
	June	224	224	92	101	641	30.5
	July	157	174	102	102	535	25.5
	August	93	132	107	92	424	20.2
	September	56	89	52	69	266	12.7
	October	55	78	48	48	229	10.9
	November	39	80	50	50	219	10.4
	December	41	83	28	42	194	9.2
1973	January	53	88	42	42	225	11.2
	February	38	77	39	63	217	10.8

Source: Adapted from Robert L. DuPont and Mark H. Greene, "The Dynamics of a Heroin Addiction Epidemic," *Science* 181 (1973): 716–722.

Figure 6.3
Heroin-Related Deaths, District of Columbia: 1971–1982

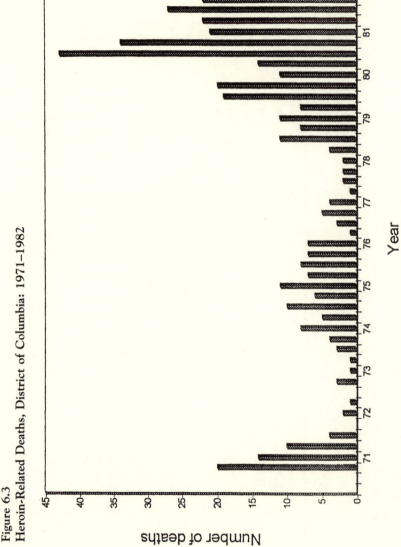

Source: A. James Ruttenberger and James L. Luke, adapted from "Heroin-Related Deaths: New Epidemiologic Insights,"
Science 226: (1984): 14–20.

Figure 6.4
Number of Crime Index Offenses: Washington, D.C., 1960–1972

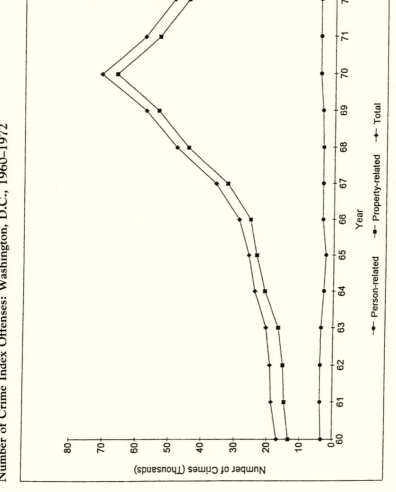

Source: Adapted from Robert L. DuPont and Mark H. Greene, "The Dynamics of a Heroin Addiction Epidemic," *Science* 181 (1973): 716–722.

The property-crime rates in the District of Columbia fell earlier than the other measures of heroin addiction prevalence. Before NTA opened its doors, several other sources were making methadone available in the District in late 1969, including the Department of Corrections pilot program, a few private physicians, and a local activist organization called Blackman's Development Center (BDC), headed by the charismatic and highly visible Hassan Jeru-Ahmed, a self-styled colonel. When NTA began operations in early 1970, there was a dramatic increase in the availability of methadone in the city. NTA grew to more than two thousand active patients by July 1970.

Suddenly, in late 1969 and early 1970, the heroin scene in the District of Columbia changed. Addicts in large numbers had alternatives to continued heroin use. Heroin addicts with big habits, the ones most likely to commit many income-generating property crimes, were some of the first patients to enter NTA treatment. The increase in police activity, which began at the same time NTA started its efforts, had synergistic effects with the NTA's heroin addiction treatment. The highly visible police buildup made it more difficult to be a criminal heroin addict in the years after 1969. Heroin became less available after 1969, giving an added incentive to addicts to enter NTA treatment.

The private physicians who had flooded the city's streets with methadone in late 1969 and early 1970 were cited for flagrant drug law violations, and BDC closed operations in 1972, so that by that year, NTA was virtually the only source of methadone in the city. Many of NTA's admissions in 1970 and 1971 had previously been treated at BDC and by the private physicians who sold methadone prescriptions to heroin addicts.

The incidence of new heroin use fell sharply soon after 1970. The massive increase in heroin treatment by NTA played an important role in reducing the prevalence of heroin use, because addicts had alternatives to continued heroin use. In addition, increased law enforcement after 1969 reduced the availability of heroin. The heroin problem in the early 1970s was so huge and so visible that potential new heroin users could clearly see that heroin use most often led either to prison or to the morgue. This evidence dampened enthusiasm for new heroin experimentation among vulnerable youth. Heroin was no longer just another drug in Washington by 1972 (Craig and Brown 1975).

DEMOGRAPHICS IN THE DISTRICT

The demographic context of the D.C. heroin epidemic included major population trends (DuPont 1973a, 1394–1402). Heroin addiction disproportionately affected the baby boom generation. Less widely recognized was the steady increase in black migration from North Carolina and other parts of the South to the District from the 1920s through the 1960s. The population of the overall Washington metropolitan area had been about 25 percent black since about 1900, and the proportion stayed fairly constant through the 1970s. However, the percentage of the population that was black in the District itself rose from 35 percent in 1950 to 71 percent in 1970. The rise in the proportion of black people did not trigger the heroin epidemic. Rather, the national heroin epidemic hit Washington in 1970 as these demographic changes were occurring.

This shift in racial makeup was not associated with a reduction in living standards in the city. The median education of adult blacks in D.C. rose from 8.8 years of schooling in 1950 to 11.4 years in 1970. The number of black adults who had completed college rose from ten thousand in 1950 to twenty-two thousand in 1970. The rise in median income for black families, adjusted for inflation to 1970 dollars, rose from $2,200 in 1950 to $6,500 in 1970. Most black migrants from the South to the District of Columbia improved their living conditions, in terms of both education and income. The unemployment rate in the District was generally low during the post-Depression migration. In 1970 the unemployment rate for black men aged twenty to fifty-nine was 4.5 percent; for black women it was 3.6 percent.

The migration from the South and the baby boom combined to push the number of people between the ages of sixteen to twenty-one—the age most vulnerable to beginning heroin use—from sixty-five thousand in 1960 to eighty-six thousand in 1970. This shift reflected an increase in this age group from 8.5 percent of the population to 11.4 percent in a decade. This age segment of the population of the District of Columbia rose by 32.2 percent in the decade after 1960. The black population aged fifteen to twenty-four rose from 56,000 in 1960 to 105,000 in 1970, an 88 percent increase. The rise in the youth population was matched by a proportionate fall in the percent of the population of adults between the ages of twenty-five and fifty-five, the age group most responsible for the behavior of youth between fifteen and twenty-four. This drop in the proportion of mature adults reflected the relatively low birth rates nationally in the 1920s and 1930s.

An impact of the baby boom generation on D.C. during the late 1960s had been foreshadowed earlier in the decade. The dropout rate from junior high school began to rise sharply in 1962, peaked in 1964, and fell to a lower level after 1969. A similar phenomenon was seen in senior high schools, where the trend to more dropouts began a few years later and peaked in 1968. The rate of serious crime, disproportionately associated with the population of young men, began to rise in the District of Columbia in 1966 and peaked in 1969.

The D.C. baby boomers entered the labor market at a time of economic prosperity. The unemployment rate in the District in the 1960s was about 3 percent, substantially lower than the corresponding national rates. Embedded in this overall statistic was the rate of unemployment for blacks aged sixteen to twenty-one, which rose steadily, from about 8 percent during the early 1950s to 16 percent for males and 20 percent for females in 1970, still low by national standards at that time (Wilson and DuPont 1973, 91–98).

The NTA data on drug problems in the District of Columbia between 1970 and 1973 were detailed in many professional publications (see, e.g., DuPont 1971; DuPont and Katon 1971; Brown et al. 1972; Greene and DuPont 1974, 545–50; Greene and DuPont, eds., 1974, 1–56; Greene, Brown, and DuPont 1975; Greene, Nightingale, and DuPont 1975).

THE NATIONAL CONTEXT

Like Washington, D.C., most other large cities in the United States had heroin epidemics with incidence of new heroin use peaking between 1969 and 1971. Some smaller communities experienced epidemics having peaks of new heroin use a few years later. While the rises of heroin use and crime in other cities were similar to those in D.C. (as were the population changes), the fall of heroin use in the District of Columbia was earlier and sharper than in other communities. It should be noted that no other city had the comprehensive level of data on heroin use that was available for the District. In D.C. the active heroin user population (prevalence of heroin addiction) declined from about fifteen thousand in 1970 to about two thousand in 1973. New York City's methadone program was the only other program in the country on the scale of NTA in the early 1970s. New York showed a similar peaking of admissions to heroin addiction treatment in mid-1972 as well as similar patient characteristics (Newman et al. 1973). There is also a review of early NTA experiences with a comparison to national crime figures (Massing 1998a).

LESSONS LEARNED FROM THE NTA EXPERIENCE

Data from NTA during its first three years can be used to answer the two public health questions posed at the beginning of this chapter. First, it proved possible and affordable to implement a large-scale, communitywide treatment program for heroin addicts. Second, a treatment-based approach to the heroin epidemic benefited not only individual addicted patients but also the entire community.

The success of NTA opened new ground in American drug policy by showing that large-scale heroin addiction treatment could be delivered on a cost-effective basis and that treatment had positive communitywide effects on rates of both addiction and crime. How much of the benefit in terms of reduced heroin use and reduced crime experienced in Washington in the early 1970s was attributable to addiction treatment, separate from the dynamics of the epidemic, increased police activity, and curtailment of heroin supplies as a result of international activities, remains unknown. However the credit for the sharp fall in heroin addiction is divided between treatment and law enforcement, it is hard to look at the data that are available for that period in the District of Columbia and not conclude that heroin addiction treatment produced dramatic positive results. The experience in the District of Columbia in the early 1970s validated a balanced strategy including both treatment and law enforcement, which became the national policy in 1971. The policy shift brought hope to hundreds of thousands of addicted people nationwide.

NTA data provided a profile of the modern heroin epidemic. These data showed who was addicted to heroin and offered important insights into the dynamics of the heroin epidemic. For example, the data demonstrated that heroin addiction was both an endemic and an epidemic disorder, primarily of young men in the inner city, and, further, that the disease often persisted for decades in individual addicts. We also learned that heroin addiction released its victims for longer or shorter periods of time in response to changes occurring in the community. As treatment became widely used, the rates of drug use fell sharply. The rate of heroin use (prevalence) was responsive to easily accessible and effective drug abuse treatment. The profile of people caught in this heroin epidemic in the District of Columbia was linked to the demographic bulge known as the baby boom and to urban migration over the past decades.

Despite this impressive result, after 1973 the political will to treat heroin addicts dissipated. The resulting loss of public support led directly to a reversal of the positive heroin prevalence trends. In short order D.C. experienced a renewed rise in heroin overdose deaths and in crime. The epidemic rise in the incidence of new cases of heroin use in the District of Columbia, however, did not recur after 1973. The prevalence of heroin use within the epidemic cohort was responsive to the availability of treatment initiatives in the early 1970s and to the relative lack of treatment options in the city in later years. Neither the rise in heroin overdose deaths in the late 1980s to levels higher than those seen before the buildup of NTA nor the corresponding rise in crime rates sparked a renewed commitment to addiction treatment in the District of Columbia. The big rise in the prevalence of heroin use after 1973 was the result of large numbers of people who first used heroin in the 1966–69 period stopping between 1971 and 1973, only to resume use after 1973.

The tidal wave of crack cocaine in the late 1980s and early 1990s had a devastating impact on this epidemic population, as did the AIDS epidemic, which began about the same time. These developments made NTA's simple formula (use methadone to treat heroin addiction to benefit both addicts and the community) appear to be out of date, even quaint. The rise in marijuana use since the 1970s also demonstrated that NTA's focus on heroin addiction was a two-edged sword. On one hand, this specific focus permitted an effective response to a single drug problem—intravenous heroin addiction. On the other hand, coupled with its controversial reliance on methadone, NTA's highly focused strategy sowed the seeds of its own loss of political viability, as evidence of success against heroin addiction after 1973 reduced support for the District's treatment efforts.

LESSONS FROM THE EARLY NTA EXPERIENCE

First, the drug problem is bigger than the heroin problem. Even the best focused responses to heroin use are unsustainable politically over time without a commitment to deal with other illegal drug problems as well.

Second, when good news comes about drug addiction, the political support necessary to mount an effective treatment response evaporates. Only a growing addiction problem appears able to command the political support needed to create and maintain a large-scale community response to addiction. Addiction treatment was the first and most important casualty of this sudden fall of political support for anti-drug efforts after 1973. The major rise of crack cocaine and of crime in the District of Columbia in the late 1980s (including a terrifying rise in the murder rate) showed that even a sharply rising drug-crime problem did not lead to a heightened commitment to addiction treatment. In contrast to the early 1970s, in the late 1980s there was no vision and no organized effort in the District of Columbia to harness the political uproar caused by the renewed rise in crime and addiction.

Third, lasting recovery from addiction depends on prolonged participation in the twelve-step programs such as Alcoholics Anonymous, Narcotics Anonymous, and Al Anon. NTA in the early 1970s was oblivious to this fundamental reality of addiction and recovery (DuPont and McGovern 1994).

The ebb and flow of public support for addiction treatment in the District of Columbia in the late 1960s and early 1970s appeared to be an expression of a larger cycle of tolerance and intolerance for illegal drug use that has been identified in the nation as a whole (Musto 1999). As the drug problem worsens, the determination to reduce drug use builds. Once the tide is turned on drug use, the anti-drug fervor wanes, and anti-drug efforts abate. This change produces tolerance for illegal drug use, setting the stage for a renewed rise in the rates of drug use. A similar alternating pattern has been seen in youths' marijuana use, where the ebbs and flows of youthful "disapproval" of marijuana use are inversely related to the use rates in American teenagers (Johnston 1998).

One prominent criticism of NTA's early successes was that the program's supporters were motivated merely by a desire to reduce crime. Skeptics argued that NTA's goal was not medical, but merely "political." To NTA supporters, reducing crime obviously was a medical goal. Crime has many victims, including the criminals themselves, who suffer terribly not only from imprisonment but also from the lifestyles they adopt. Reducing crime was an important public health goal, and to the extent that medical treatment of heroin addicts helped to achieve this goal, successfully reducing crime was a public health triumph. The vagaries of American politics in the 1970s did not see it that way. Crime reduction was commonly thought to be a right-wing, mean-spirited, even racist and inhumane political goal. Besides, liberals had bigger concerns. They wanted to end poverty and racism by attacking the "root causes" of heroin addiction.

Even conservatives, while remaining strong advocates of crime reduction, were troubled by using addiction treatment to achieve this goal. Addiction treatment was expensive, often not successful, and appeared to "coddle" addicts rather than holding them accountable for their illegal behaviors (crime and drug use). Heroin addiction treatment, especially the use of methadone, remains today what it was in 1970, largely a political orphan.

NTA's political support rested heavily on the goal of crime reduction. When the crime rate in the District of Columbia fell in the early 1970s, the support for many anti-crime programs, including NTA, fell even more dramatically. Treating addicts as a primary public health objective was both a boost to NTA and, in its later years, a major source of its decline. The uncharted boundaries of the human problems covered by the magic word *addiction* bedeviled later drug abuse treatment and prevention strategies. Policymakers were left to consider a tangle of separate but related behavioral problems, none of which had clear-cut treatments resembling the way methadone treated heroin addiction. Their ability to create effective political leverage for addiction treatment vanished.

THE FUTURE OF TREATMENT

The first three years of the Narcotics Treatment Administration provided a clear picture of the modern heroin epidemic and demonstrated that it was possible to intervene with addiction treatment to reduce the prevalence of heroin use in an entire community.

Clear peaks of incidence (new use) of heroin were found in 1950 and 1969, with the latter peak being larger than the former. The prevalence of heroin use was shown to be responsive to treatment and other interventions, while the incidence of use fell quickly, as vulnerable youth learned about the devastating consequences of heroin addiction. Substantial (but lesser) endemic heroin initiation also occurred.

NTA was a model that led directly to a change in national drug policy. After NTA's success, treatment was added to law enforcement to produce a balanced national drug-abuse strategy. However, NTA's treatment initiative in the District of Columbia was not sustained, as controversies about both its methods and goals consumed early optimism.

A question for the future is whether a dedicated effort at addiction treatment, more broadly focused, could be developed and sustained. Further, would the results of a major addiction treatment effort be seen in changes in communitywide rates of drug use and resulting communitywide problems, such as crime? Finally, a related question was raised by the NTA experience. If a treatment-based strategy worked for individuals and the community, could the political will to support it be maintained, or does success in treating addicts in an entire community inevitably lead to political and financial abandonment?

REFERENCES

Alsop, Stewart. 1972a. "The Road to Hell." Newsweek, March 6.
———. 1972b. "To Save Our Cities." Newsweek, April 10.
American Journal of Public Health Supplement. 1974. 64. (December).
Baum, David. 1960. Smoke and Mirrors: The War on Drugs and the Politics of Failure. Boston: Little, Brown.
Brown, Barry S., Urbane F. Bass III, Susan K. Gauvey, and Nicholas J. Kozel. 1972. "Staff and Client Attitudes Toward Methadone Maintenance." International Journal of the Addictions 7, no. 2: 274–55.
Courtwright, David T. 1982. Dark Paradise: Opiate Addiction in America Before 1940. Cambridge, Mass.: Harvard University Press.
Craig, Starlett R., and Barry S. Brown. 1975. "Comparison of Youthful Heroin Users and Nonusers from One Urban Community." International Journal of the Addictions 10, no. 1: 53–64.
DuPont, Robert L. 1971. "Profile of a Heroin-Addiction Epidemic." New England Journal of Medicine 285: 320–24.
———. 1972. "The District of Columbia Experience Treating Heroin Addicts." Public Management 54: 7–9.
———. 1973a. "Where Does One Run When He's Already in the Promised Land?" Proceedings of the Fifth National Conference on Methadone Treatment, 1394–1402. Washington, D.C.: National Association for the Prevention of Addiction to Narcotics.
———. 1973b. "Coming to Grips with an Urban Heroin Addiction Epidemic." Journal of the American Medical Association 223: 46–48.

———. 1973c. "Perspective on an Epidemic." Washington, D.C.: Washington Center for Metropolitan Studies, October 29. Unpublished data.

———. 1997. *The Selfish Brain: Learning from Addiction.* Washington, D.C.: American Psychiatric Press.

DuPont, Robert L., and Mark H. Greene. 1973. "The Dynamics of a Heroin Addiction Epidemic." *Science* 181.

DuPont, Robert L., and Richard N. Katon. 1971. "Development of a Heroin-Addiction Treatment Program: Effect on Urban Crime." *Journal of the American Medical Association* 216: 1320–24.

DuPont, Robert L., and Doris Layton MacKenzie. 1994. "Narcotics and Drug Abuse: An Unforeseen Tidal Wave." In *The 1967 President's Crime Commission Report: Its Impact Twenty-five Years Later.* Edited by John A. Conley. Highland Heights, Ky.: Academy of Criminal Justice Sciences; Cincinnati, Ohio: Anderson Publishing.

DuPont, Robert L., and John P. McGovern. 1994. *A Bridge to Recovery: An Introduction to 12–Step Programs.* Washington, D.C.: American Psychiatric Press.

DuPont, Robert L., and Eric D. Wish. 1992. "Operation Tripwire Revisited." In *Annals of the American Academy of Political and Social Science* 521: 91–111.

Gladwell, Malcolm. 1998. "Just Say 'Wait a Minute.'" *New York Times Book Review,* December 17.

Greene, Mark H., Barry S. Brown, and Robert L. DuPont. 1975. "Controlling the Abuse of Illicit Methadone in Washington, D.C." *Archives of General Psychiatry* 32, no. 2: 221–26.

Greene, Mark H., and Robert L. DuPont. 1974. "Heroin Addiction Trends." *American Journal of Psychiatry* 131.

Greene, Mark H., and Robert L. DuPont, eds. 1974. "The Epidemiology of Drug Abuse, Part 2." *American Journal of Public Health* 64.

Greene, Mark H., James L. Luke, and Robert L. DuPont. 1974. "Opiate Overdose Deaths in the District of Columbia: Heroin-Related Fatalities." *Medical Annals of the District of Columbia* 43: 175–81.

Greene, Mark H., S. L. Nightingale, and Robert L. DuPont. 1975. "Evolving Patterns of Drug Abuse." *Annals of Internal Medicine* 83: 402–11.

Johnston, L. D. 1998. "1998. 'Monitoring the Future' Study Results." Press release of Office of National Drug Control Policy. Ann Arbor: University of Michigan, Institute for Social Research, December 18.

Jonnes, Jill. 1996. *Hep-Cats, Narcs, and Pipe Dreams: The History of America's Romance with Illegal Drugs.* New York: Scribner.

Kozel, Nicholas J., and Robert L. DuPont. 1977. *Criminal Charges and Drug Use Patterns of Arrestees in the District of Columbia.* National Institute on Drug Abuse Technical Paper, DHEW Publication no. (ADM). Washington, D.C.: NIDA.

Lowinson, Joyce H., J. Thomas Payte, Edwin Walsitz, Herman Joseph, Ira J. Marion, and Vincent P. Dole. 1997. "Methadone Maintenance." In *Substance Abuse : A Comprehensive Textbook.* Edited by Joyce H. Lowinson et al. Baltimore: Williams and Wilkins.

Massing, Michael. 1998a. "Nixon Had It Right: A 70's Project Showed Drug Treatment Works." *Washington Post*, November 8.

Massing, Michael. 1998b. *The Fix*. New York: Simon and Schuster.

Musto, David F. 1999. *The American Disease: Origins of Narcotic Control*. 3d ed. New York: Oxford University Press.

Newman, Robert G., Sylvia Bashkow, and Margot Cates. 1973. "Analysis of Applications Received by the New York City Methadone Maintenance Treatment Program During Its First Two Years of Operation." In *Proceedings of the Fifth National Conference on Methadone Treatment*, 802–10. Washington, D.C.: National Association for the Prevention of Addiction to Narcotics.

Presidents' Commission on Crime in the District of Columbia Report. 1966. Washington, D.C.: U.S. Government Printing Office.

President's Commission on Law Enforcement and Administration of Justice. 1967a. *Task Force Report: Narcotics and Drug Abuse*. Washington, D.C.: U.S. Government Printing Office.

———. 1967b. *Task Force Report: Narcotics and Drug Abuse. Annotations and Consultants' Papers*. Washington, D.C.: U.S. Government Printing Office.

Ruttenberger, A. James, and James L. Luke. 1984. "Heroin-Related Deaths: New Epidemiologic Insights." *Science* 226 (5 October): 14–20.

Wilson, James Q., and Robert L. DuPont. 1973. "The Sick Sixties." *Atlantic Monthly*, October.

7

Generational Trends in Heroin Use and Injection in New York City

Bruce D. Johnson and Andrew Golub

In this chapter we examine the epidemiology of heroin use and abuse in New York City during the past century. Our review is based on over thirty-five years of ethnographic and survey research on heroin and other drug use in New York City, a major center for heroin use, and upon a reading of the broader scientific literature. The ethnographic research provides detailed and holistic insights into the social context in which heroin use takes place and the heroin careers of individuals. The survey research identifies the prevalence and general persistence of use.

Household surveys indicate that heroin use has been confined to an extremely small portion of the population in the past twenty years or longer; from 1979 through 1998, not much more than 1 percent of the general population ever reported any lifetime use of heroin (SAMHSA 1999). The study of heroin use was greatly enhanced with the founding of the Arrestee Drug Abuse Monitoring (ADAM, formerly DUF, or Drug Use Forecasting) program in 1987. The prevalence of heroin use has been much higher among arrestees, due to heroin's illegality and the lifestyles of many people who use it. Consequently, ADAM provides systematic data about trends in heroin use among a population of particular interest to policymakers. The ADAM data are used in this chapter to reconstruct the epidemiology of heroin use among Manhattan arrestees over a twelve-year period.

Overall, heroin and injection drug use in America have followed epidemic-like waves of popularity. These waves have been situated according to geographical location, historical period, and subcultural activity. In particular, heroin use has been primarily concentrated in certain high-risk populations in some cities (but not others) and has impacted certain birth cohorts, referred to here as the Heroin Injection Generation, much more than others. Many members of this Heroin Injection Generation have persisted for twenty and even thirty years in their use. At the hundredth birthday of the synthesis of this substance, this generation comprises the "bolus" of heroin consumers in the 1990s, especially among inner-city residents who tend to get in trouble with the law. While several highly publicized claims about a new wave of heroin use occurred in the 1990s, actual increases in use have been isolated geographically and are quite small in comparison to the great tsunami that swept the country in the 1960s and early 1970s.

THEORETICAL CONSTRUCTS

This section introduces several key constructs employed in studying the social context of substance use, abuse, sales, and distribution, particularly as they relate to heroin.

Drug Subcultures and Conduct Norms

Many sociologists, as well as anthropologists, philosophers, policy analysts, and members of other disciplines, focus on understanding the culture within which individuals operate. Culture is a particularly rich and holistic construct. UNESCO captured this complexity in the official definition adopted at the second World Conference on Cultural Policy in Mexico City in 1982:

> Culture ought to be considered today the whole collection of distinctive traits spiritual and material, intellectual and affective, which characterize a society or social group. It comprises, besides arts and letters, modes of life, human rights, value systems, traditions and beliefs. (Schafer 1998, 28)

Substance use and abuse are cultural or, perhaps more accurately, subcultural (that is, affecting a subset of the larger population within a specific cultural context) phenomena. The particular substances an individual uses and the significance of that use depend heavily on when, where, and among whom ingestion takes place. Quite often, some groups of individuals will encourage the use of various substances at the same time that others living in the same city strongly proscribe use.

With regard to heroin use, individual behavior is the most proximal concern, although it is values, symbols, and beliefs that define and help interpret the context for these behaviors. In this regard, a principal focus of ethnographic drug research is the accurate identification of the various conduct norms that serve as "rules of behavior" governing individual conduct and interactions with others in a situation (Wolfgang and Ferricuti 1967; Johnson 1973, 1980; Johnson, Dunlap, Maher 1998). These norms are often extremely context-specific. In studying substance use, the focus is on those conduct norms associated with drug use, abuse, sales, and distribution which combine to create drug subcultures.

The conduct norms of drug subcultures govern how individuals and small groups use heroin (inhale, smoke, snort, inject), whether and how it is shared, the implicit bartering process behind the purchase and sharing of drugs, how consumers think and talk about heroin, and involvement in heroin sales and distribution (Johnson et al. 1985). For example, during 1968, high-risk youths in New York City reported (that is, the conduct norms encouraged) "snorting heroin" and were enthusiastic about "mainlining" heroin for the best highs; they happily initiated their friends and relatives to such use. Active consumers of heroin constituted the core of this heroin subculture and often organized much of their life and resources around their consumption of heroin. (Note: Many heroin subculture participants also engage other drug subcultures, such as cocaine and marijuana, although others do not [Johnson 1973, 1980; Johnson et al. 1985]). Thirty years later, high-risk youths report conduct norms promoting near-total avoidance of heroin, needle use, and "junkies"; they express a preference for marijuana over heroin (Golub and Johnson 1999). Among the relatively few heroin-using youths in New York City, "sniffing " (the conduct norms imply consumption of smaller amounts than when "snorting") predominates over injection (Hamid et al. 1997; Furst et al. 1998, 1999; Friedman et al. 1998).

An Epidemic Model

Different drugs tend to go in and out of favor. Much prior literature (Becker 1963, 1967; Golub and Johnson 1999; Hamid 1992; Johnston 1991; Musto 1973, 1974; Reinarman and Levine 1997) has suggested that the ebb and flow in the popularity of any particular drug tends to follow a pattern similar to a disease epidemic. We distinguish four distinct phases to any drug epidemic: incubation, expansion, plateau, and decline.

A drug epidemic typically starts slowly, with use confined to a small group, in an incubation phase. Once it gains broader acceptance, an expansion phase begins, and the drug's popularity spreads rapidly, following the S-shape pattern common to a wide range of diffusion phenomena (Rogers 1995). The dramatic initial growth is physically limited by the number of people willing to try the drug. Once most of these individuals become users, or at least have had the opportunity to do so, a drug epidemic enters a plateau phase, during which it continues as an important drug of choice for many persons. Youths who come of age during the plateau phase tend to use the current drug(s) of choice, if any. A drug epidemic typically enters a decline phase as youths coming of age become less inclined to initiate drug use and/or do not remain regular users. This decline might be the result of another diffusion process, in which the idea that the drug is "bad" spreads within the broader population and, more important, also spreads among the high-risk youths. This new attitude among youths foretells the eventual end of a drug epidemic. However, overall declines are generally slow in coming, as many existing users persist in their habits—even after a drug's broader appeal has diminished among the young.

The term "drug epidemic" emphasizes the underlying nature of substance use as a social contagion (Musto 1991, 1993). The term "drug era" stresses how use is situated within the broader social context of a long historical period. The evidence presented below indicates that two major "heroin eras" occurred in America in general, and in New York City specifically, having their peaks (which are identified primarily as the expansion and plateau phases) from about 1900 to 1920 and 1965 to 1974. We refer to these periods as the First Heroin Era and the Heroin Injection Era respectively, the latter title identifying the primary mode of heroin consumption during the second historical period.

Birth Cohort and Drug Generations

The epidemic model emphasizes that the choice of drugs an individual tends to use depends heavily on which drugs were popular at the time he or she came of age. Thus, a drug epidemic is especially associated not only with a particular time but also with a particular birth cohort, individuals born in the same year or group of years. Individuals who came of age during the peak of the Heroin Injection Era are referred to as the Heroin Injection Generation. The evidence presented below indicates that relatively few individuals born in the years before or after this generation used heroin, especially by injection.

Political Scapegoating

The existence of multiple and conflicting subcultures in New York City (and throughout America) has led to extended culture clash, because different groups held diametrically opposing views about use of a particular substance. One manifestation of this animus has been an almost continuous scapegoating of drugs and drug abusers for more than eighty years by mainstream figures and institutions, especially politicians and the media (Musto 1973, 1994; Morgan 1981; Courtwright 1982, 1992a, 1992b, 1996, 2002; King

1972; Gray 1998). Heroin use has been blamed for the broader problems facing society, including crime, violence, reduced productivity, poverty, family tension, and declining morality.

In response to this conflict, government agencies have prohibited heroin, made its possession and sale illegal, passed laws imposing harsh penal sanctions, devoted extensive police resources to arresting heroin users and sellers, supported courts in prosecuting heroin cases, and incarcerated hundreds of thousands in jails and prisons for long sentences. Heroin users and sellers have been depicted as heinous and depraved persons—the modern functional equivalent of demons and witches. Yet these individuals endure, because their subcultures and social networks view heroin use as an important symbol, a central part of their identity, and a pleasurable activity. Additionally, regular heroin use typically leads to physical dependence, often rendering individuals unable to stop even if they want to.

The politically popular trend has been for legislators to advocate or pass laws, sanctions, and terms of imprisonment designed to "get tough" on heroin users and sellers. Numerous persons attending the 100 Years of Heroin Conference—including the former highest-ranking agency and public policymakers in the drug abuse field—had their reputations crucified in the political arena and the press because they were branded as "soft" (or not "tough enough") on heroin users and sellers.

HEROIN USE PRIOR TO 1940

In this section, we will briefly summarize the early spread of heroin use for nonmedical purposes. (For more detailed discussion of the historic origins of heroin use, see the Introduction and chapter 1 in this volume.)

Terry and Pellens (1928) indicate that in the late 1800s, morphine and other opiates were legal, easily obtained, and widely used for medical purposes by professionals, for self-medication of various ailments by consumers, and for pleasure. The Bayer Pharmaceutical Company invented heroin in 1898 and initially marketed it as a powerful cough suppressant. However, no legal restrictions stopped individuals from using it for other purposes and, indeed, conduct norms developed that encouraged the recreational use of opiates. The existing opiate users, and especially the numerous morphine injectors, rapidly discovered that heroin was "better" because it gave a quicker "high" (Terry and Pellens 1928; Courtwright 1982a; Johnson 1975a). Heroin could be legally purchased without prescription, and in large quantities (that is,100 mg. or more). Most consumers probably inhaled ("snorted") the pharmaceutically pure heroin.

This led to the First Heroin Era, approximately 1900–1920. Unfortunately, far too little is known about what happened to persons who became addicted to heroin at that time. During the early part of the century, anti-drug norms pushed drug use into underground subcultures. Paramount among the institutional changes was the passage of the Harrison Act (1914), which established the licensing and prescription system still used for dispensing drugs at the end of the century (see Musto 1973, 1999; Courtwright 1986a, 1992a, 1992b, 2002).

In response to the Harrison Act, during and after World War I several jurisdictions established narcotic clinics as a way to legally provide heroin to addicts. The New York City Health Department established the nation's largest narcotic clinic at Worth Street; it provided maintenance doses of heroin and morphine to opiate users from 1918 to 1920 (Musto 1973, 278–84). While this clinic (and other maintenance clinics) had many organizational problems, several distinguished scholars contend that they were quite effective in following a public health paradigm for disease treatment and prevention (Brecher 1972; Musto 1973; Musto and Ramos 1981; Waldorf et al. 1974; Courtwright 2002; Gray 1998).[1] The clinics dispensed limited doses of heroin or morphine on a regular basis at relatively low cost to active addicts, and thereby both contained the activities of users and prevented widespread sale of heroin by illicit heroin peddlers.

However, others judged these programs as outright "failures" because they did not lead existing users to desist completely from heroin use. This assessment took hold as the claims of moral entrepreneurs (Becker 1963, 1967) gained ascendancy with the formation of the Prohibition Bureau and later the Federal Bureau of Narcotics (the latter led by Harry Anslinger). These agencies actively interpreted the Harrison Act as prohibiting maintenance of active addicts, and threatened and/or initiated prosecutions of several physicians for doing so. By 1922, almost all clinics providing heroin or morphine to addicts were closed, including those in New York City (Musto 1973, 1993, 1994).

Despite clear rulings by the U.S. Supreme Court in the Berman (1921) and Linder (1926) cases that the Harrison Act was a tax act and did not forbid physicians from prescribing heroin or opiates to addicted patients, almost all prescribing physicians have avoided prescribing heroin or morphine on a long-term, outpatient basis to active heroin addicts since the mid-1920s.[2] Likewise, from the 1920s to the 1950s, heroin abusers in New York City had virtually no access to drug treatment other than questionable forms of detoxification (Courtwright et al., 1981, 1989).

Scapegoating of heroin and addicts became popular. After a moral crusade led by Hobson (Musto 1973), federal law was changed in 1924 to prohibit legal manufacture and sale (even via prescription) of heroin in America. Since 1924, the federal government has held an "abstinence only" policy toward heroin. Federal (and most state) policy is limited to promoting complete abstinence from heroin and other illegal drugs), suppressing use, and punishing those who do use, and especially those who sell, heroin. Public health efforts (for example, drug treatment, alternatives to incarceration, methadone maintenance, needle exchanges, and other such programs) have been distinctly secondary options, and often have conflicted with the government's continued commitment to an abstinence policy and a primary reliance upon criminal justice approaches.

In this intolerant climate, however, illegal heroin sales have flourished. Informal heroin transactions had been known in New York City even when legal, prior to 1914. However, illegal supply mechanisms became more important and commonplace with implementation of the Harrison Act in 1914 and picked up even more after the city's maintenance clinics were closed in the 1920s. The heroin seller (or "dope peddler") became a minor but constant fixture in New York's underground economy.[3] Perhaps as a result of being forced underground, illicit sales of the less potent drugs opium and morphine declined as heroin became the primary opiate available. Heroin sellers conducted virtually all business through private networks; selling occurred mainly in homes, businesses, or other private locations—rarely in public locales. The heroin peddler was constantly targeted, scapegoated, and punished by city, state, and federal governments. But punishments for heroin possession and sale in the period 1930–50 were modest; indeed, relatively few persons were incarcerated, especially compared to later in the century.

HEROIN USE AMONG MANHATTAN ARRESTEES, 1987–97

At this point, it is appropriate to have a short break before continuing the history of heroin use, in order to discuss the importance of new technology to the study of heroin's history. In the late twentieth century, America underwent an information revolution, with both growth in the power of computers and dramatic expansion in their use for storing massive amounts of information. An important part of this revolution was the creation of annual survey programs to monitor shifts in attitudes and behaviors over time. This information provides a powerful archive for, and can add much greater precision to, historical analyses of social phenomena, such as drug use trends. This section documents the epidemiology behind the Heroin Injection Era by using data from one ongoing survey, the ADAM program, for the years 1987–1997. In the next section, epidemiological theory and ethnographic insights will be combined to reconstruct the nature and timing of the Heroin Injection Era. Then we will briefly extend this New York City analysis to twenty-three locations across the country that were in the ADAM program as of 1997.

The current ADAM program, which spends over a million dollars per year and operates at several dozen sites nationwide, had its humble beginnings in a few small research projects in Washington, D.C., and Manhattan in the early 1980s (Wish et al. 1984; Wish and Johnson 1986). These projects demonstrated that arrestees would agree to cooperate with a drug use survey and that substance use was widespread among arrestees. A unique feature of the ADAM program is asking arrestees to provide a urine sample that is subsequently tested for illegal drugs. All arrestees are asked to participate voluntarily, are informed of the purpose of the project, and are assured that the information they provide will be used for research purposes only and will not affect their individual cases. Upward of 90 percent of arrestees approached have agreed to participate. Starting in 1987, the National Institute of Justice (NIJ) launched the Drug Use Forecasting (DUF) program at a few sites. By 1997 the program had expanded to twenty-three locations, including all U.S. cities with a population in excess of one million, as well as several smaller cities to provide geographic diversity (NIJ 1997, 1998).[4] In 1998, the program evolved and expanded into the Arrestee Drug Abuse Monitoring (ADAM) program with plans to increase to up to seventy-five sites between 1998 and 2001 (NIJ 1999).

Manhattan was the first DUF/ADAM site and has been in the program since the second quarter of 1987. On a quarterly basis, project staff collect self-reports of drug use and urine specimens from about 250 adult male and 100 adult female arrestees.[5] The urine specimens are tested for ten illegal drugs. The opiate-positive urinalysis results document heroin use during the past three days. Urinalysis results provide critically important information that often documents current use of drugs—even when arrestees deny any current or even lifetime use.

The current study employs ADAM-Manhattan data from 13,674 arrestees interviewed from 1987 to 1997. During this period, the demographic characteristics of arrestees were generally quite stable. (See table 7.1 for a summary.) Over half were African-American, just over a quarter were Hispanic, and an eighth were white. About 28 percent were female.[6] Over half were ages twenty-one to forty at arrest. Three-quarters were single/never married. Only about an eighth reported being married. A third had less than a high school education.

A third of ADAM-Manhattan arrestees self-reported lifetime heroin use, a fifth self-reported heroin use in the preceding thirty days, and a fifth were detected as opiate-positive.[7] Cocaine was even more popular. Two-thirds were detected as cocaine-positive, although only half self-reported lifetime cocaine use and 43 percent reported lifetime crack use. Lifetime marijuana use was reported by 71 percent, but only 23 percent were detected as having used marijuana in the preceding thirty days.

A fifth reported lifetime injection of drugs. Ethnographic evidence indicates that most heroin injectors preferred "speedballs," heroin and cocaine powder combined into a mixture and consumed in the same injection. East Harlem heroin abusers studied in 1980–82 used cocaine on about half as many days as they used heroin; a quarter of their drug expenditures involved cocaine purchases (Johnson et al. 1985). In short, the "heroin injection generation" (born 1945–59) was also heavily involved in cocaine use via injection and, later, crack smoking as well. Virtually no New York arrestees or street drug users engage in cocaine injection only, without also injecting heroin.

The trend in heroin-use measures (lifetime use, use in past thirty days, lifetime injection, and being opiate-positive at arrest) fluctuated somewhat—but not greatly—during 1987–97 (see figure 7.1). Youthful arrestees (ages 18–20) had levels of heroin use about a third or less than those of the adults. The general directions of trends for all four heroin indicators are similar, despite some year-by-year fluctuations. All four indicators of heroin use among youthful arrestees declined by almost half between 1996 and 1997 (also see Johnson, Thomas, and Golub 1998).

Birth year was highly correlated with these heroin indicators. About half of ADAM-Manhattan arrestees born between 1945 and 1954 self-reported lifetime heroin and injection use; and over a quarter were detected as opiate-positive at arrest during the period 1987–99 (see figure 7.2). For all heroin indicators, the proportions of heroin users declined steeply across birth years.

Among arrestees born in the 1960s, about 20 percent were detected as opiate-positive at arrest, and only 10–20 percent reported lifetime injection of drugs. Among arrestees born after 1971, under 12 percent were detected as opiate-positive, and only about 5 percent reported injection drug use. Fewer than 5 percent of those born between 1977 and 1979 reported lifetime heroin use or were detected as heroin users. Fewer than 5 percent of arrestees born after 1971 (and thus young adults in their twenties during the 1990s) self-reported any lifetime injection experience. This analysis of heroin use as a function of birth year strongly suggests that the Heroin Injection Generation was composed primarily of persons born shortly after World War II and closely corresponded to the baby boom generation, born between 1946 and 1964. The two five-year birth cohorts with greatest involvement in heroin and drug injection were 1945–49 and 1950–54.

Members of these birth cohorts reported having first initiated heroin use primarily during the 1960s and early 1970s (see figure 7.3). Among arrestees from the 1950–54 birth cohort, 14 percent began heroin use and drug injection in their late teens (in 1965–69), and an additional 11 percent began injection in their early twenties (1970–74). Nearly as many arrestees from the 1945–49 birth cohort initiated drug injection early on, but did so mainly

Table 7.1
Demographic Characteristics, Charges, and Drug Use
Indicators: ADAM-Manhattan Arrestees, 1987–97
(N = 13,674)

	%	Count
Gender		
Male	72	9,780
Female	28	3,894
Race/Ethnicity		
Black	54	7,392
White	13	1,836
Hispanic	30	4,042
Other/Missing	3	404
Five-Year Birth Cohorts		
1900–44	4	574
1945–49	5	664
1950–54	11	1,505
1955–59	18	2,449
1960–64	24	3,257
1965–69	20	2,786
1970–74	12	1,706
1975–79	5	679
1980–84	0	54
Age at Arrest		
<18	4	592
18–20	8	1,160
21–25	18	2,466
26–30	22	2,954
31–35	20	2,700
36–40	14	1,906
41–45	8	1,039
46–50	3	448
51+	3	409
Interview Year		
1987	4	513
1988	9	1,187
1989	10	1,351
1990	10	1,320
1991	10	1,376
1992	8	1,045
1993	11	1,508

Table 7.1 *Continued*

	%	Count
1994	8	1,069
1995	10	1,430
1996	11	1,437
1997	11	1,438
Marital Status		
Single	74	10,131
Married	13	1,838
Sep/Wid/Div	12	1,698
Education		
No H.S. Degree	34	4,653
H.S. Grad	24	3,282
In H.S.	3	428
G.E.D.	5	725
Some College	12	1,656
College Grad.	6	802
Missing	16	2,128
Top Arrest Charge		
Drug Possession	13	1,730
Drug Sales	6	806
Robbery	11	1,548
Burglary	6	866
Larceny	20	2,673
Violent Index	14	1,871
Other Income	7	979
Other Series	9	1,190
Other	15	2,011
Drug Use Indicators		
Opiate Positive	20	2,740
Inject Ever (SR)	21	2,611
Heroin Ever (SR)	33	4,553
Heroin—30 days (SR)	20	2,737
Cocaine Positive	66	9,055
Coc Powder Ever (SR)	49	6,638
Crack Ever (SR)	43	5,913
Marijuana Positive	23	3,159
Marijuana Ever (SR)	71	9,671
Other Drug Positive[a]	8	984

[a]Includes only 1989–97 subsample.
(SR) Self Reported

Figure 7.1
Heroin Use Indicators by Interview Year, 1987–1997

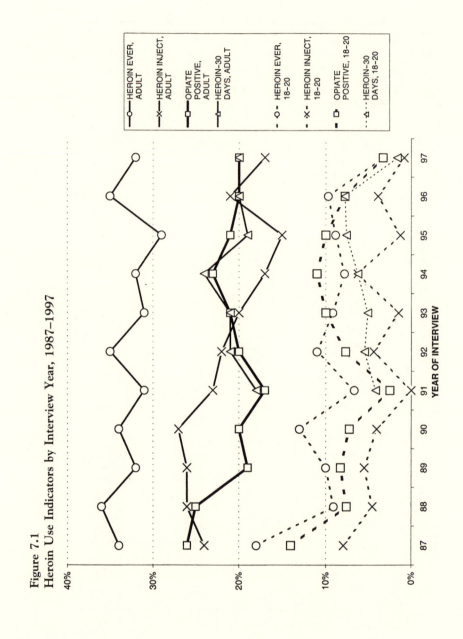

Figure 7.2
Heroin Use Indicators by Birth Cohorts, 1900–1979

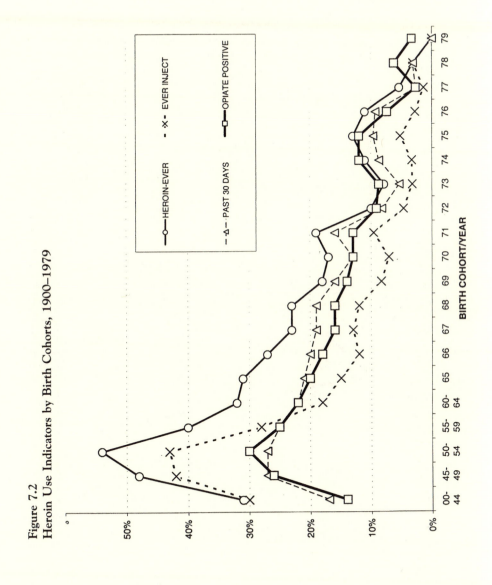

Figure 7.3
Variation in Years of First Drug Injection by Birth Cohorts: ADAM-Manhattan Arrestees
born 1945–1959, 1970–1974

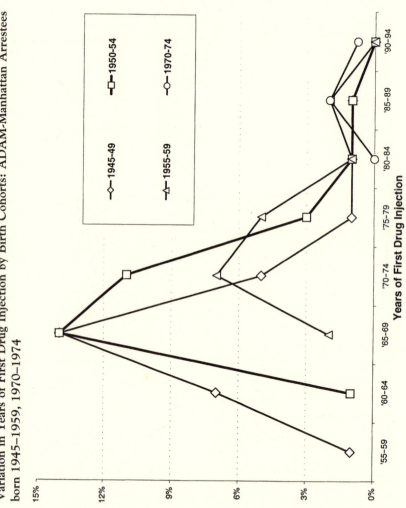

in their twenties (in the late 1960s). Among arrestees in the 1955–59 birth cohort, a smaller percentage (only 7 percent) initiated injection drug use in their teens and an additional 5 percent in their early twenties.

In stark contrast, only 2 percent of arrestees born between 1970 and 1974 began injection drug use in their teens, and only an additional 1 percent in their early twenties. While some proportion of heroin users desisted from heroin use and injection, a very sizable proportion of inner-city heroin users among the birth cohorts born between 1940 and 1959 continued heroin use and injection throughout their adult lives.[8] These birth cohorts also have commonly been found among those with heroin-use problems who come to the attention of the police, other criminal justice agencies, emergency rooms, drug treatment programs, and social service systems. Most likely, this birth cohort will comprise a substantial portion of all heroin users and injectors in future years.

Inner-city African-American youths born in the 1970s—many of whom are children or grandchildren of heroin abusers—appear to have developed strong conduct norms against heroin use and systematically to have avoided heroin use and injection during their teens and twenties (Furst et al. 1998, 1999). This avoidance of heroin and injection drug use by high-risk, inner-city youths occurred despite the facts that (1) they often had parents, relatives, or neighbors who regularly used or injected heroin; (2) heroin was easily available in their neighborhoods; (3) retail heroin was of higher potency than that available twenty years before; (4) heroin sellers routinely attempted to entice new customers by mixing heroin with cocaine or marijuana; (5) some nonheroin-using youths engaged in heroin sales; and (6) needle exchanges were available to provide clean "works" to persons requesting them. Recent ethnographic studies and HIV-research projects in New York City have had major difficulty finding subjects under age twenty-one from minority inner-city backgrounds who used heroin, especially via injection (Hamid et al. 1997; Johnson, Dunlap, and Associates 1998). Even among the relatively few heroin consumers in the youthful generation, most reported preferring to "sniff" heroin and also avoided the use of needles (Hamid et al. 1997).

A more comprehensive analysis of the ADAM-Manhattan data revealed three important "drug generations" among Manhattan arrestees.[9] Arrestees born in successive years exhibited important changes in their preferred drugs of regular use. In large measure, these "drug" generations may be defined by where the lines in figure 7.4 diverge sharply by birth year. The Heroin Injection Generation can be identified by the increased use of heroin among arrestees with birth years in the 1940s and early 1950s. After the 1954 birth year, the graph indicates strong and steady declines in injection drug use and heroin use. The Cocaine/Crack Generation can be identified as arrestees born between 1950 and 1967, because on average over half of them reported crack

Figure 7.4
Key Drug Use Indicators by Birth Year: ADAM-Manhattan Age 18+, 1987–1997, n = 13,084

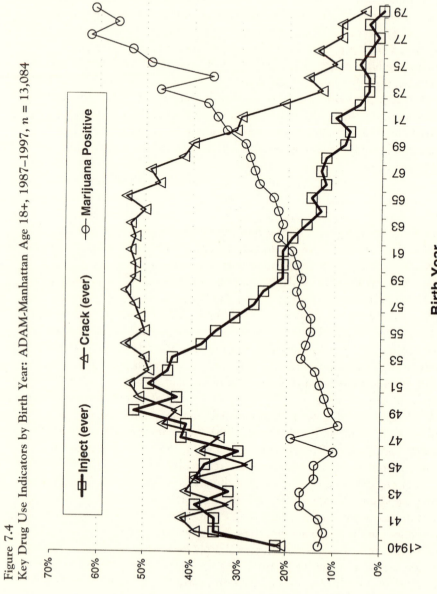

Birth Year

use over the eleven-year reporting period. Steady declines in reported crack use start with the 1967 birth year. The Blunts/Marijuana Generation can be identified by the increasing rate of detected marijuana use starting with the 1970 birth year, but especially among those born 1975 and later.

THE HEROIN INJECTION ERA IN NEW YORK CITY

The epidemiological data from the ADAM program can now be combined with the theoretical constructs developed earlier—and with ethnographic, historical, treatment, and HIV/AIDS data—to reconstruct the Heroin Injection Era and its associated consequences in New York City, especially in Manhattan. In many respects, the following represents a relatively clear example of a well-documented "drug epidemic" that has continued for nearly forty years.

Incubation Phase

The lowest levels of heroin use and sales in the twentieth century occurred during World War II (Musto 1973), probably as a result of three major factors. First, the "first heroin generation" (those who, for the most part, were born between 1880 and 1900 and who began when heroin was still legal) had given it up, or died, or grown too old to be active in the heroin culture. Second, the government had drafted, provided military training to, and mobilized millions of teenage men, so the number of young males in New York at high risk for heroin initiation was dramatically reduced, compared to before or after the war. Third, war efforts disrupted existing routes of illegal heroin importation, making heroin hard to obtain. But World War II and the immediate postwar years also generated conditions that set the stage for the Heroin Injection Era.

The second epidemic of heroin use had a particularly strong impact on blacks and other ethnic minorities who had recently migrated to New York. During and soon after World War II, hundreds of thousands of rural and small-town individuals and families (especially African-Americans) emigrated from the American South and Puerto Rico to New York City. Previously excluded from wage jobs, such immigrants found employment in many war factories or in low-wage jobs, or benefited from expansion of the city's welfare system. Especially after the end of the war, these migrants, along with millions of other Americans, began having children. The postwar "baby boom," those born between 1945 and 1964, contributed disproportionately to the Heroin Injection Era. As the following story will show, many of the youths growing up in America's inner cities at this time fared poorly in achieving conventional status measures (education, employment, stable families); many became involved in criminality, drug use, and illegal drug sales (Iiyama et al. 1976; Johnson et al. 1990).

With the end of the war, heroin trade routes were reestablished, and heroin selling resumed. Within certain subcultural contexts, heroin developed a very positive image, especially among many jazz musicians and their hangers-on (Courtwright 1999; Brown 1965; Thomas 1967). These pursuits of pleasure increased in peacetime. For most of the 1950s, however, heroin selling primarily occurred in private places, and almost never in public locations (see Malcolm X and Haley 1966; Brown 1965). Heroin buyers had to "know someone," get a referral to the seller, and make transactions in private spots (typically, an apartment or bar). This soon would change.

Expansion Phase

In the 1960s, supplies of heroin became more regularized, and some dealers gained control over the distribution of heroin in key localities. Nicky Barnes controlled heroin distribution and many heroin sellers in Harlem; he became an important presence in the community. Persons who grew up in Harlem in the 1960s remember Barnes and his associates organizing block parties, giving "loans" that did not need repayment, and helping when times were tough.[10]

In the 1950s and early 1960s, many youths from low-income families became members of fighting gangs like those immortalized in the musical *West Side Story* (see Schneider 1999). In 1963 a former colleague, Ed Preble, was hired as an outreach worker to help prevent gang warfare in East Harlem. He was not too successful. But in the following year he noticed that his gang contacts were suddenly lethargic and had little interest in fights and rumbles (Preble 1975). He soon discovered the reason: heroin. In a very fundamental way, the conduct norms governing the status-seeking behavior of such inner-city teen groups had changed from being a leader of a gang with members interested in fighting and rumbles to just being "cool" (Finestone 1965). The consumption of marijuana and heroin was initially viewed as "cool," because it gave a great high, providing euphoria and escape from the tensions of life. Youthful social groupings soon reorganized around the continuing pursuit of heroin and the sharing of funds, drugs, and needles, rather than around gang membership and fights.

Heroin users introduced others to the conduct norms of the heroin subculture (Johnson 1973; Johnson et al. 1985; Johnson, Thomas, and Golub 1998; Johnson et al. 2000).

Those conduct norms included the following. Heroin is the greatest high. Continue using it again and again. At an early stage, don't use often enough to become addicted. Snorting doesn't provide a good high any longer. Try skin-popping (injection under skin). Heroin injection is even more effective than snorting or skin-popping to get high and to get the most from every precious bag of heroin. Speedballs (cocaine mixed with heroin) are a great way to go "fast then slow." Learn a variety of needle-injection practices and rituals. Share heroin and needles when you don't have enough heroin. Go to a shooting gallery to inject heroin. Rent works for injection. Pay the gallery owner by giving him a taste of your heroin. Borrow and engage in various hustles to raise money to purchase heroin. Locate the seller with the best bag of heroin. Engage in various crimes to generate income to purchase heroin. Sell heroin to make good money and maintain a large habit. Learn various strategies for avoiding police, reducing probability of arrest or lengthy penal sanctions. Learn how to avoid others who would rob by force or steal your drugs or money (see Johnson et al. 1985; Johnson et al. 2000).

Plateau Phase

A relatively new heroin subculture emerged in the mid-1960s, especially among inner-city minority youths. Persons who sold heroin achieved considerable status in the heroin-using community (Preble and Casey 1969). Heroin sellers began conducting their business in public places (streets, parks, bars, and so forth). While initiates to heroin typically began by experimenting with "snorting" it, most rapidly moved on to "skin popping" (injecting heroin under the skin), and often to "mainlining" (injecting into a vein) on a daily basis within a year.

During the plateau phase of the Heroin Injection Era, users often devoted their entire economic and criminal activity to obtaining money to support their habits and to consuming heroin. Doing so provided a sense of purpose and meaning that was denied to them in conventional society (Preble and Casey 1969; Johnson et al. 1985). Their daily activities ranged from quasi-legal hustles to a variety of nondrug crimes, and numerous drug sales or distribution roles to obtain money or drugs. Their time was spent in chasing the best bag of heroin, locating a safe place to inject, sharing with other users, avoiding police, finding "free" food, shelter, and clothing, and conning others into sharing drugs or needles. On the average, they injected heroin about twice per day, but they often had days with no heroin use (Johnson 1984; Johnson et al. 1985).

The processes described above and the conduct norms regarding heroin use (Preble and Casey 1969) prevailed in New York City among groups of African-Americans, Puerto Ricans, and many low-income whites (Preble and Johnson 1978). Heroin addiction, mainly via injection drug use, became widespread in minority communities in the 1965–74 period. Youths growing up in minority and low-income neighborhoods were quite likely to initiate heroin use and, if they became addicted, to remain regular heroin users. The primary period when a very substantial proportion initiated heroin was 1965–1969. Studies found that nearly a quarter of the young men in Manhattan had experimented with heroin, and about half of these had developed addictions (see O'Donnell et al. 1976; Clayton and Voss 1981; Brunswick and Boyle 1979; Boyle and Brunswick 1980). As discussed above, the ADAM-Manhattan data suggest that many of them remained active heroin users throughout most of their adult lives.

Heroin selling became an important occupation in inner-city New York in the 1970s. Sellers developed their own "bag markings" to distinguish their "brand" of heroin from those sold by competitors (Goldstein et al. 1984). The number of heroin sellers in public places began increasing; some blocks became major "drug supermarkets" where hundreds of buyers and sellers came to conduct business. While the quality of the heroin was quite poor (1–5 percent, averaging 2 percent), the retail price of a street heroin bag remained at $10 throughout the 1960s and 1970s (Johnson et al. 1985). Many heroin sellers discovered that cocaine selling could be very profitable, as demand for cocaine was increasing in the late 1970s. Some began selling cocaine but not heroin.

This epidemic of heroin use did not go unnoticed by conventional society, nor was it condoned. The dramatic increases in youthful heroin use and addiction became both a public concern and a major media story in the 1960s. Numerous articles in the *New York Times* and other newspapers and magazines sensationalized the heroin problem, effectively transforming heroin and its users into scapegoats for the many difficult social problems that emerged during this decade. As the heroin subculture was becoming institutionalized, a wide range of other crises took police resources away: the civil rights movement, the Black Power movement, the Vietnam War protests, and widespread use of marijuana, psychedelics, and other illicit drugs. The occurrence of "civil disorders" (which were serious in New York City but less severe than in other major cities) meant that many police officers were reassigned to maintain order (National Advisory Commission on Civil Disorders 1968).

Nevertheless, a wide variety of social and governmental responses to heroin abuse were initially developed, and some became institutionalized. The origins of the current drug treatment system were clearly established between 1964 and 1970—and continued to the end of the century. The various treatment modalities included detoxification, outpatient counseling, methadone maintenance, and therapeutic communities. City, state, and federal governments launched a variety of initiatives designed to control heroin abusers and sellers (Massing 1998; Krogh 2002; Jaffe 2002; White 2002).

New York Governor Nelson Rockefeller instituted three major initiatives to address the heroin problem in New York State. First, in 1965 he estab-

lished the Narcotic Addiction Control Commission (NACC), which provided for criminal and civil commitment to "jail-like" treatment facilities
(Waldorf 1971, 1973; Lipton and Johnson 1998); most of these were con-
verted from prisons, or built to "treat" the growing population of heroin addicts. Second, New York State began to allocate substantial sums of state
dollars to drug treatment; federal dollars, which came later in the 1970s, only
supplemented state funding. NACC provided state funding for drug treatment
slots in community-based treatment programs. The Addiction Services
Agency was established to administer these treatment funds in New York City.
State and federal funds supported a growing number of drug-free outpatient
programs and residential drug treatment programs, particularly therapeutic
communities. Third, in the early 1970s, Governor Rockefeller became unhappy with NACC performance; and as a would-be presidential candidate
he sought to establish himself as "very tough on drug sellers."[11] In 1973 he
proposed the Rockefeller Drug Law, which gave life sentences to heroin and
narcotic sellers (even those who sold small amounts).

Two of these major Rockefeller-era programs were subsequently judged as
failures. Both in effect were politically inspired efforts that scapegoated heroin
users and especially heroin sellers. These laws constituted efforts by the majority (and an aspiring politician) to impose their "abstinence" standards and
morality upon the heroin-addicted minority. In 1965 proponents of the
NACC facilities anticipated that they could successfully transform heroin
users into "drug-free" citizens. However, their optimism was misplaced. Very
few of the thousands of heroin addicts sent to such facilities remained abstinent after departure from these criminal commitment facilities (Lipton and
Johnson 1998). The NACC criminal and civil commitment facilities were
closed in 1976 (Waldorf 1971, 1973, 1988). Civil and criminal commitment
facilities were also established by the federal government and by the state of
California—and closed in the 1970s.[12]

Governor Rockefeller equally optimistically claimed that heroin sellers
would be deterred from future sales by the prospect of mandatory life sentences. Virtually every authority doubted that claim even as the legislation
was being passed in 1972; a subsequent evaluation found little or no deterrent effect on heroin sellers by 1976 (New York City Bar Association 1976).
However, approximately five thousand sellers were sentenced to life terms
and as of 1999 were still New York State prisoners. Efforts to repeal mandatory life sentences under this law have not passed the state legislature (New
York Times 1999).

In New York City, Mayor John Lindsay supported Dr. Vincent Dole and
Marie Nyswander in establishing methadone maintenance programs (Dole
and Joseph 1978; Lowinson et al. 1997); for many years, the New York
City Health Department operated the largest such program in the world.

Methadone maintenance provided ongoing treatment for heroin addicts. By the early 1970s, these programs served about thirty thousand clients a year.[13] Heroin detoxification became popular with addicts seeking to reduce the cost of their habits (Alling 1992; Gray 1998). Therapeutic communities such as Synanon and Phoenix House were established as an important, albeit expensive, option for helping addicts develop a drug-free lifestyle. Much research (DeLeon 1984, 1997; DeLeon et al. 1972) has established the efficacy of these programs both for keeping drug users out of the criminal justice system and for helping them become drug-free (Anglin and Perrochet 1998; GAO 1990). In many respects, community-based treatment programs were more successful than criminal justice programs because they were not so heavily committed to abstinence from heroin as their primary goal, but instead stressed a set of intermediate goals (much less heroin or drug use, lower crime levels, family stability, employment) that made client progress more incremental and achievable for treatment participants. On the other hand, treatment dropout rates have been and remain very high.

In the period 1974–78, New York City government experienced near-bankruptcy, caused by years of heavy borrowing to support social services. Thousands of city workers, including police, firemen, and teachers, were laid off and the city's entire social service network was seriously damaged. New York City got out of the drug treatment business and closed the Addiction Services Agency. A single New York State agency (then called Office of Drug Abuse Services) managed contracts directly with local treatment agencies in New York City. The police also retrenched and concentrated drug enforcement resources on high-level sellers. The police department and other jurisdictions had instituted the era of "professional policing," whereby officers avoided situations that could lead to their extended involvement with, and possible corruption by, criminal drug sellers (Kelling and Coles 1996; Wilson 1963).

In the period 1960–80, the heroin subculture in New York City developed a unique institution known as the "shooting gallery." Galleries were either apartments or sections of abandoned buildings where users came to inject heroin (Johnson et al. 1985). Usually they were run by a heroin-addicted proprietor who "rented" works (injection equipment). Addicts came to galleries to have a safe place to inject heroin, enjoy the high, and socialize. The proprietor was paid in cash, in heroin, or by sharing an injection (having a "taste" of the addict's shot). Needle-sharing (and reuse) practices at these shooting galleries propelled the widespread transmission of Hepatitis B and C and of the HIV/AIDS virus among addicts in the early 1980s (Des Jarlais et al. 1994, Shilts 1987). At this time, a sharp turn in conduct norms against heroin use, especially via injection, began among younger persons in those neighborhoods.

Decline Phase

Only in the mid-1970s did the proportion of inner-city young adults initiating use of heroin begin to decrease (Boyle and Brunswick 1980; Clayton and Voss 1981; Hunt and Chambers 1976), signaling the beginning of the decline phase of the heroin epidemic (see figure 7.3). The ebbing, or slow decline, of heroin abuse in New York is primarily the product of fewer youths initiating heroin, regular use, or injection use. Such youthful "avoidance" of heroin use (and of crack smoking), and especially its injection, was a fundamental part of inner-city youth culture and conduct norms in the 1990s. Youths may choose to sell heroin to "junkies," as a way of making money; but heroin use itself is to be avoided. The downward trend in heroin initiation means that fewer "replacements" are available when someone from the Heroin Injection Generation dies or goes "off heroin" for a while. Consequently, the overall pool of regular heroin abusers continues to shrink. While the availability, retail price ($10 a bag), and quality (40–70 percent pure) of heroin sold on the streets of New York City rarely have been better, heroin use and injection are slowly "ebbing" (Johnson, Thomas, and Golub 1998; Johnson, Golub, and Dunlap 2000).[14]

Whereas youths became uninterested in heroin, the large pool of heroin abusers who initiated during the Heroin Injection Era (1965–74) persisted in their habits into the adult and later adult years of their lives. Such consumers constitute the most visible representatives, and remain the "core," of the heroin problem in New York City. Even a quarter-century later, in 1987–99, the majority of arrested heroin injectors reported an age at first heroin use that corresponds to initiation in the late 1960s or early 1970s (see figures 7.1 and 7.4; Golub and Johnson 1999). For most of the 1970s, 1980s, and 1990s, estimates of the number of active (in the past year) heroin users ranged between 200,000 and 250,000 in New York City (Frank et al. 1978; Johnson and Muffler 1997).

During the last quarter of the twentieth century, members of the Heroin Injection Generation (those born 1940–54) matured into adulthood, approaching or passing their fiftieth birthdays—if still living. A modest number of active heroin users die each year from causes including homicide and drug overdose, as well as alcoholism, heart disease, and other chronic conditions (Joseph and Appel 1985; Joseph et al. 1983). In the late 1970s, HIV/AIDS was added to this list of hazards. Studies (Des Jarlais et al. 1989, 1994; Stoneburner et al. 1988) in the 1980s showed that approximately a third to half of New York City's injection drug users had HIV; persons who regularly injected at shooting galleries had higher HIV rates. In the 1980s, injection drug use and needle sharing was the second leading means of HIV transmission in New York City (after male-male sex [Shilts 1987]). In short, early death is an important component of the ebbing of the Heroin Injection Era cohort, especially among those who remained persistent heroin abusers during their adulthood.

While some heroin injectors are dying at young ages, of equal interest is that others have survived so long. Extensive ethnographic information has documented that many heroin injectors consider themselves "controlled users"; they may be physically addicted, but they are able to keep their consumption in check (Brunswick 1988; Brunswick and Titus 1998; Brunswick and Messeri 1992; Brunswick et al. 1992; Waldorf and Bernacki 1981; Nurco 1998). One technique these heroin users employ for asserting their control is to occasionally cut back on their use or even to go "off" heroin for a while. This leads to intermittent use of heroin across an adult career (Anglin and Perrochet 1998, Nurco 1998). Some intermittency in heroin use is involuntary. Users may be off heroin while incarcerated, because heroin is unavailable to them or because it is overly expensive (G. H. Hunt and Odoroff 1962; Lipton et al. 1991).

Some individuals use detoxification or methadone maintenance to provide a respite from their heroin habit (Milby 1988). When they subsequently return to heroin use, they can achieve a better high with less heroin. Still others may use drugs other than heroin and thus go off heroin for a while. Particularly in the 1980s, many heroin addicts added crack smoking to their polydrug habits; a few of these spent all their funds on crack, so effectively got "off heroin" (Johnson et al. 1994). Some switched to alcohol, which is both legal and cheaper than heroin (Preble and Miller 1977). Thus, persons who are "intermittently off" heroin probably constitute a substantial proportion of the Heroin Injection Generation at any given time.

The social perception and scapegoating of heroin users eased considerably in the 1980s with the rise of cocaine and crack use. The preferred drugs among inner-city youths in New York became cocaine powder (1972–85) and then crack (1984–89). Many publications (Johnson et al. 1995; Golub and Johnson 1994b, 1996, 1997) and news media (Reinarman and Levine 1997) have documented the rapid expansion of powder cocaine snorting. Although cocaine snorting was scientifically evaluated as relatively less harmful than heroin in the 1970s (Waldorf 1998), political changes in the 1980s led to the development of "tougher" policies against it. With the advent of "crack" or "rock" cocaine in the mid-1980s, what was effectively a "new" drug in epidemiological terms (Johnson et al. 1994; 1995) became the substance which society and government scapegoated and punished most severely. Public concern about heroin abuse declined somewhat as crack became the "monster" drug in the public eye and the governmental policy scapegoat (Belenko 1993; Brownstein 1996; Hartman and Golub 1999; Reinarman and Levine 1997; Chepesiuk 1999).

The large pool of persons who began heroin injection in the 1965–74 period continued to be the main group of heroin users in New York in the 1990s. Even though early death has been common (due to overdose, homicide, alcoholism, and HIV/AIDS) among this cohort, and although many are intermittently "off" heroin (due to incarceration, treatment, cross-addiction, and voluntary abstinence), the Heroin Injection Generation's substance abuse and offending behavior is continually documented by analyses of populations seeking treatment. So the "ebbing" of the heroin epidemic continues as a very slow decline in New York City at the beginning of the twenty-first century.

HEROIN USE IN OTHER CITIES

New York City was an important epicenter of the Heroin Injection Era. The timing and intensity of the era varied elsewhere throughout the country (Chein et al. 1964; Hunt 1973; Hunt and Chambers 1976; Rittenhouse 1977; Inciardi and Harrison 1998). Heroin use in the general population is substantially less than among arrestees. In responses to the National Household Survey on Drug Abuse (SAMSHA 1999), persons born in the years 1945 through 1959 generally report among the highest proportions of lifetime heroin use (Golub and Johnson 1998).[15] Less than 3 percent of the householders contacted report any lifetime use; much less than 1 percent report heroin use during the past thirty days—a far lower rate than among arrestees.

Data from the ADAM program in twenty-three cities permit comparative documentation of the magnitude of the heroin problem among those individuals who tend to get in trouble with both drug abuse and the law across the country. The national ADAM data provide strong support for the argument that the Heroin Injection Era was centered in New York City, confirming other ethnographic and historical data. From 1987 through 1997, the majority of the other twenty-two ADAM jurisdictions never had any substantial heroin use among arrestees; most had rates below 10 percent. In those jurisdictions with significant (over 10 percent) heroin prevalence, a pertinent finding is that younger arrestees are much less likely to be heroin users than those born in 1945–59. Heroin-related findings for the twenty-three ADAM/DUF locations participating during 1987–97 are summarized in Map 7.1. For the most part, levels of detected heroin use among arrestees were low nationwide, with a few exceptions on a city-by-city, as opposed to regional, basis. In most ADAM locations, identified with asterisks, fewer than 10 percent—often much less (1–3 percent)—of arrestees were consistently detected as opiate users.

Rates of heroin use among arrestees were considerably higher, relative to national levels, in several major cities. A few locations (Detroit, Los Angeles, Manhattan, San Antonio, San Diego, Washington, D.C.), marked by squares in Map 7.1, exhibited a slowly declining rate of detected opiate use, as some individuals born in the 1940s and 1950s and initiators of heroin use in the 1960s and 1970s continued their use in the 1980s and 1990s. Arrestees from the Heroin Injection Generation constituted a continually decreasing proportion of the total arrestee population. Interestingly, the decline in heroin use in Chicago did not start until the mid-1990s. Three ADAM sites— Portland (Oregon), New Orleans, and St. Louis—exhibited a modest resurgence in heroin use (indicated by upward arrows) among arrested youths coming of age in the 1990s. The overall picture is that heroin use and abuse are quite rare among arrestees (and in emergency rooms) in most metropolitan areas of the United States; heroin is relatively more common only in a few, widely distributed metropolitan areas.[16]

HEROIN IN NEW YORK CITY ACROSS THE TWENTIETH CENTURY

The history of heroin use and attempts to control it strongly suggest that the conduct norms of the heroin subculture exert a far more powerful influence on heroin users than do government edicts and criminal justice initiatives. New York City has experienced two major and relatively distinct eras of heroin use: one peaking during 1900–1920, the other from 1965 to 1974. Each was characterized by an initially explosive growth in heroin use and development of pro-heroin conduct norms among user groups; this was followed by a slow ebbing, as powerful norms against heroin use developed among youths while existing users persisted with their habits. Those in the "bolus" of heroin abusers within each generation often persisted in heroin use across much of their adulthood. The continued decline of heroin injection (as well as crack smoking) among Manhattan arrestees born in the 1960s and 1970s was a major, and a most astonishing, gain for public health in the 1990s, and should continue in the next decade.

Rather than wait for a heroin era to run its course, historically America has chosen to intervene heavily to stop heroin use and sales. Since the beginning of the twentieth century, the American government for the most part steadfastly has pursued an ideologically driven policy against opiate users. Abstinence from heroin (and other illicit drugs) is vigorously promoted as the primary option to be supported and advanced by government agencies. The history of American opiates policy is characterized by pointed rhetorical declarations about the evils of heroin (or other drugs) and the morally noble importance of abstinence as *the* goal of public policy. These policy initiatives most often (a) ignore the many lessons from history and science that such policies have not "worked" before and often have created substantial

Map 7.1
Trends in Detected Opiate/Heroin Use among ADAM/DUF Arrestees Nationwide, 1987–1997

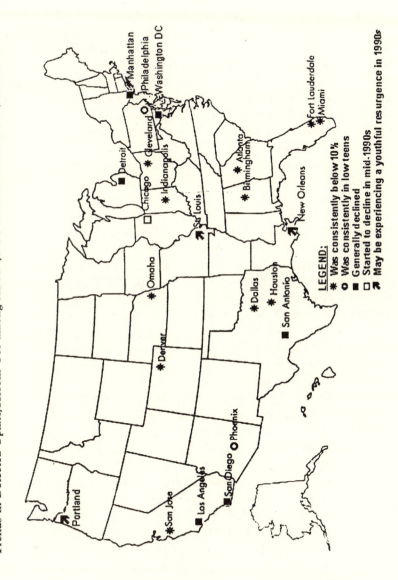

LEGEND:
* Was consistently below 10%
○ Was consistently in low teens
■ Generally declined
□ Started to decline in mid-1990s
↗ May be experiencing a youthful resurgence in 1990s

problems, (b) create new expectations and problems for a variety of agencies whose staffs must impose these policies on unwilling heroin users and sellers, and (c) create new hardships upon the targeted population, who consequently devise new strategies for avoiding the enforcement of such policies.

American politicians and policymakers have learned that promoting abstinence from heroin and other drugs is a "morally correct" position that may contribute to political or professional advancement. The rhetoric of abstinence promotion is easily stated (although often factually incorrect or misleading); scapegoating of users and of those pictured as sympathetic to users can be extensive; legislation designed to punish users is not difficult to pass; large amounts of public funds can be appropriated and new institutions can be developed to enforce the abstinence goal or to punish those caught evading it. The main lesson is that the majority can "legislate the morality of abstinence."

In their century-long pursuit of the abstinence ideal, agents of the federal government often have ended, prevented, or undermined local initiatives that followed public health models for responding realistically to the relapsing condition of heroin abuse. During the twentieth century, New York City had the nation's largest heroin problem and attempted a range of remedies. Few other cities experienced a "heroin problem" until the 1960s. No other city has ever had as many heroin addicts as New York City. Due to the magnitude of its heroin problem and to its long liberal tradition, New York has been a leader in innovative approaches to drug abuse and often has developed new policies that the federal government closed or seriously constrained.

Especially in the second half of the twentieth century, American politicians and the public resolutely supported—and extensively funded—"tough" criminal policies toward those possessing or selling heroin, despite extensive documentation that criminal justice "solutions" (a) do very little to reduce the magnitude of the heroin problem, (b) rarely achieve "abstinence" among heroin users after release from custody, and (c) are unable to target the harshest sentences upon well-documented "traffickers."

The enthusiasm for harsh punitive policies directed at heroin sellers among the American public and politicians is extraordinary in Western societies. In many respects, the clear failure of public policies such as civil/criminal commitment or life sentences are far more spectacular than the alleged "failure" of city-run heroin/morphine maintenance clinics in the 1920s. Despite imposing "corrections-based abstinence" on thousands of heroin addicts, policymakers rarely achieved the objective of producing "ex-addicts" capable of avoiding heroin after release from custody. When the amorphous policy of "deterrence" or "abstinence" from heroin use is documented as unsuccessful, however, the goal often shifts to "lock them up and throw away the key."

Legislation and institutions established with one set of purposes now are used in support of a very different set.

The history of heroin use in New York City in the twentieth century suggests that no medication, no form of drug treatment, and no criminal justice punishment approach has been developed that can ensure that even a small proportion of heroin addicts become abstinent and remain abstainers for the remaining years of their lives. The vast majority of heroin addicts entering detoxification, treatment, or correctional institutions will not remain permanently abstinent from heroin.

Government officials and policymakers need to read the trends in heroin use and the history of substance abuse treatment and control with great care in order to devise a more humane and rational policy for the twenty-first century. Despite massive funding, the government's ability to create abstinence among heroin users and stop illicit heroin selling is even more remote in 1999 than when New York's morphine maintenance clinics were closed in 1920. On the other hand, only if a resurgence in heroin use begins to occur among newer cohorts or among new subpopulations, and a new Heroin Injection Era develops, is heroin likely to reemerge as a major problem. The best long-term prognosis in 1999 is that as the number and proportion of current long-term heroin users/injectors born in the postwar years reach their fifties and sixties, they will begin to die of natural causes and also will commit fewer crimes leading to arrest. If these predictions are correct, the Heroin Injection Era in New York City will continue its slow decline and will eventually sputter to an end about 2025.

ACKNOWLEDGMENTS

Data collection for this essay was supported by the National Institute of Justice for the Drug Use Forecasting program (94-IJ-CX-A013) and the Arrestee Drug Abuse Monitoring program (National Institute of Justice and Abt Associates (OJP-98C-001).

Research was supported by grants from the National Institute on Drug Abuse (5 ROI DA05126-08, 5 ROI DA09339-03) and from the Robert Wood Johnson Foundation's Substance Abuse Policy Research Program (033027). Additional support was provided by National Development and Research Institutes.

Points of view expressed do not necessarily reflect the positions of these funding organizations or of National Development and Research Institutes.

NOTES

1. For how similar opiate-maintenance clinics functioned fifty years later in the United States and in the United Kingdom, see Johnson 1975c; 1976. See also the review of the Swiss heroin-maintenance program in chapter 10 of this volume.

2. But there were exceptions: some doctors prescribed opiates to private patients for many years in the first half of the century (O'Donnell 1969).

3. Prostitutes and numbers runners (and, during Prohibition, bootleggers and liquor dealers) were far more numerous, visible, and important than heroin sellers in New York City's illegal economy. Street vendors selling legal goods without paying taxes were far more widespread.

4. Citations to additional reports based on data from the ADAM program are available from the program's Web site (http://www.adam-nij.net) and from the National Criminal Justice Reference Service.

5. In the third quarter of 1998, the ADAM target number of arrestees was lowered to 150 adult males and 100 females. In the third quarter of 1999 a random-sampling approach was being developed to reduce the sample sizes in Manhattan to about ninety adult males and fifty females.

6. The DUF/ADAM quotas collect sufficient samples of female arrestees in order to facilitate cross-gender comparisons. In reality, only about 15 percent of Manhattan arrestees are female.

7. Manhattan arrestees had the highest or second-highest rates of detected heroin and cocaine across all ADAM sites in the United States during every year of the 1990s (NIJ 1997, 1998, 1999). A study by Golub, Johnson, and Durrah (1999) documents the rates of detected opiate use as highest (26 percent) in the Bronx, next highest (25 percent) in Brooklyn, and third highest (21 percent) in Manhattan.

8. The proportion of these birth cohorts who desisted from heroin use cannot be estimated from DUF/ADAM arrestee data (but see O'Donnell et al. 1976; Boyle and Brunswick 1980; Brunswick 1979; Brunswick and Messeri 1992).

9. In another study (Golub and Johnson 1999), we provide more extensive documentation about each of these three generations. An earlier paper (Golub and Johnson 1997; see also Golub et al. 1996) provides extensive documentation about crack's decline and changes in crack and cocaine use in all twenty-three ADAM sites. Golub and Johnson (2001) documents marijuana's upsurge among young arrestees in most ADAM sites during the 1990s.

10. Nicky Barnes and many of his associates were a very important component of the Harlem drug scene in the 1950s and 1960s; in the 1970s Barnes and several other key operatives were arrested, convicted, and sentenced to life imprisonment.

11. Being "toughest" on the drug issue did not ensure his political success. Despite great family wealth and major campaign efforts, Rockefeller never got the Republican Party's nomination for President.

12. These "prison-like treatment facilities" were as expensive as prisons to operate. Moreover, most "addicts" preferred doing prison time (where they were not expected to change their behaviors by participating in "treatment" that confronted their lifestyle). An NACC sentence also exposed addicts to reincarceration if they absconded or began using drugs after release. Indeed, most NACC facilities were prisons before 1965 and became prisons again after 1976. The actual life and "treatments" provided by staff to inmates in these facilities probably did not change much while they were under NACC control (Waldorf 1971, 1973; Lipton and Johnson 1998).

13. In many respects, methadone maintenance programs are very similar to, and can be considered the modern descendants of, the municipally run New York City maintenance clinics of the 1918–22 period. In both, a dependence-producing drug is provided legally on a regular basis to known heroin addicts by doctors and clinic personnel. Unlike heroin and morphine, which are short-acting opiates (four to eight hours), methadone and long-acting methadone (LAAM) allow for longer periods between readministration.

14. The authors have made parallel arguments that the Crack Era (1984–89) is beginning to decline because youths are avoiding crack smoking (Golub and Johnson 1996, 1997, 1998, 1999; Johnson et al. 1995). The magnitude of early deaths due to crack and of intermittency of use remain to be documented.

15. This is not true for every survey, nor for each specific metropolitan area oversampled by NHSDA.

16. Data from the Drug Abuse Warning Network (DAWN) for 1997 on locations with over 100 heroin-related emergency room episodes per 100,000 population also suggested that heroin use is particularly concentrated in a few major metropolitan areas, including Baltimore, Chicago, Newark (N.J.), San Francisco, and Seattle. (See Office of Applied Studies 1999, table 38.)

REFERENCES

"Actions of New York State Budget." *New York Times*, August 1999.

Alling, Fredric A. 1997. "Detoxification and Treatment of Acute Sequelae." In *Substance Abuse: A Comprehensive Textbook*. 2d ed. In Lowinson et al. Pp. 402–15.

Anglin, M. Douglas, and Brian Perrochet. 1998. "Drug Use and Crime: A Historical Review of Research Conducted by the UCLA Drug Abuse Research Center." *Substance Use and Misuse* 33, no. 9: 1871–1914.

Becker, Howard S. 1963. *Outsiders: Studies in the Sociology of Deviance*. New York: Free Press.

———. 1967. "History, Culture, and Subjective Experience: An Exploration of the Social Bases of Drug-Induced Experiences." *Journal of Health and Social Behavior* 8: 163–76.

Belenko, Steven. 1993. *Crack and the Evolution of Anti-Drug Policy*. Westport, Conn.: Greenwood.

Boyle, John, and Ann F. Brunswick. 1980. "What Happened in Harlem? Analysis of a Decline in Heroin Use Among a Generation Unit of Urban Black Youth." *Journal of Drug Issues* 10: 109–39.

Brecher, Edward M., et al. 1972. *Licit and Illicit Drugs*. Boston: Little, Brown.

Brown, Claude. 1965. *Manchild in the Promised Land*. New York: Macmillan.

Brownstein, Henry H. 1996. *The Rise and Fall of a Violent Crime Wave: Crack Cocaine and the Social Construction of a Crime Problem*. Guilderland, N.Y.: Harrow and Heston.

Brunswick, Ann F. 1979. "Black Youths and Drug Use Behavior: An Epidemiological and Longitudinal Perspective on Drugs Used and Their Users." In *Youth Drug Abuse: Problems, Issues, Treatment*. Edited by George Beschner and Alfred Friedman. Lexington, Mass.: Lexington Books. Pp. 443–92.

————. 1988. "Young Black Males and Substance Use." In *Young, Black, and Male: An Endangered Species*. Edited by Jack T. Gibbs. Dover, Mass.: Auburn House. Pp. 166–87.

Brunswick, Ann F., and John Boyle. 1979. "Patterns of Drug Involvement: Developmental and Secular Influences on Age at Initiation." *Youth and Society* 11: 139–62.

Brunswick, Ann F., and Peter Messeri. 1992. "Pathways to Heroin Abstinence: A Longitudinal Study of Urban Black Youth." *Advances in Alcohol and Substance Abuse* 5, no. 3: 103–22.

Brunswick, Ann F., Peter Messeri, and Stephen P. Titus. 1992. "Predictive Factors in Adult Substance Abuse: A Prospective Study of African-American Adolescents." In *Vulnerability to Drug Abuse*. Edited by Meyer D. Glantz and Roy W. Pickins. Washington, D.C.: APA Press. Pp. 419–72.

Brunswick, Ann F., and Stephen P. Titus. 1998. "Heroin Patterns and Trajectories in an African-American Cohort, 1969–1990." In *Heroin in the Age of Crack Cocaine*. Edited by James A. Inciardi and Lana D. Harrison. Beverly Hills, Calif.: Sage. Pp. 77–108.

Chein, Isadore, et al. 1964. *The Road to H*. New York: Basic Books.

Chepesiuk, Ron. 1999. *Hard Target: The United States War Against International Drug Trafficking, 1982–1997*. Jefferson, N.C.: McFarland.

Clayton, Richard R., and Harwin L. Voss. 1981. *Young Men and Drugs in Manhattan: A Causal Analysis*. Rockville, Md.: National Institute on Drug Abuse.

Courtwright, David. 1982. *Dark Paradise: Opiate Addiction in America Before 1940*. Cambridge, Mass.: Harvard University Press.

————. 1986. "Charles Terry, *The Opium Problem*, and the Origins of American Narcotic Policy." *Journal of Drug Issues* 16: 421–34.

————. 1991. "Drug Legalization, the Drug War, and Drug Treatment in Historical Perspective." *Journal of Policy History* 3: 393–414.

————. 1992a. "A Century of American Narcotic Policy." In *Treating Drug Problems*. Vol. 2. Washington, D.C.: National Academy Press. Pp. 1–62.

————. 1992b. "Drug Laws and Drug Use in Nineteenth-Century America." In *The Constitution, the Law, and American Society*. Edited by Donald Nieman. Athens: University of Georgia Press.

————. 1996. *Violent Land: Single Men and Social Disorder from the Frontier to the Inner City*. Cambridge, Mass.: Harvard University Press.

————. 2002. "The Road to H: The First Sixty Years of Heroin in America." Chapter 1 in this volume.

Courtwright, David, Herman Joseph, and Don Des Jarlais. 1981. "Memories from the Street: Oral Histories of Elderly Methadone Patients." *Oral History Review* 9: 47–64.

————. 1989. *Addicts Who Survived: An Oral History of Narcotic Use in America, 1923–1965*. Knoxville: University of Tennessee Press.

DeLeon, George. 1984. "Program-based Evaluation Research in Therapeutic Communities." In *Treatment Research Monograph Series* no. 51. Edited by Frank M. Tims and Jacqueline P. Ludford. Rockville, Md.: National Institute on Drug Abuse.

DeLeon, George, ed. 1997. *Community as Method: Modified Therapeutic Communities for Special Populations and Special Settings.* Westport, Conn.: Greenwood.

DeLeon, George, S. Holland, and Mitchell S. Rosenthal. 1972. "Phoenix House: Criminal Activity Dropouts." *JAMA* 226: 686–89.

Des Jarlais, D. C., S. R. Friedman, D. M. Novick, J. L. Sotheran, P. Thomas, S. R. Yancovitz, D. Mildvan, J. Weber, M. J. Kreek, R. B. S. Maslansky, T. Spira, and M. Marmor. "HIV-1 Infection Among Intravenous Drug Users in Manhattan, New York City, from 1977 Through 1987." *JAMA* 261, no. 7: 1008–12 .

Des Jarlais, D. C., S. R. Friedman, J. L. Sotheran, and R. Stoneburner. 1989. "The Sharing of Drug Injection Equipment and the AIDS Epidemic in New York City: The First Decade." *NIDA Research Monograph* 80. Rockville, Md: NIDA.

Des Jarlais, D. C., S. R. Friedman, J. L. Sotheran, J. Wenston, J. Marmor, S. R. Yankovitz, B. Frank, S. T. Beatrice, and D. Mildvan. 1994. "Continuity and Change Within an HIV Epidemic: Injection Drug Users in New York City, 1984 Through 1992." *JAMA* 27: 121–27.

Dole, Vincent, and Herman Joseph. 1978. "Long-term Outcome of Patients with Methadone Maintenance." *Annals of the New York Academy of Sciences* 311 (September 29): 181–89.

Finestone, Harold. 1965. "Cats, Kicks, and Color." In *The Other Side.* Edited by Howard Becker. New York: Free Press. Pp. 281–97.

Frank, Blanche, James Schmeidler, Bruce D. Johnson, and Douglas S. Lipton. 1978. "Seeking Truth in Heroin Indicators: The Case of New York City." *Drug and Alcohol Dependence* 3, no. 5: 345–58.

Friedman, Samuel R., R. Terry Furst, Benny Jose, Richard Curtis, Alan Neaigus, Don C. Des Jarlais, Marjorie F. Goldstein, and Gilbert Ildefonso. 1998. "Drug Scene Roles and HIV Risk." *Addiction* 93, no. 9: 1403–16.

Furst, R. Terry, Richard Curtis, Bruce D. Johnson, and Douglas Goldsmith. 1998. "The Rise of the Street Middleman/woman in a Declining Drug Market." *Addiction Research* 5, no. 4: 1–26.

Furst, R. Terry, Bruce D. Johnson, Eloise Dunlap, and Richard Curtis. 1999. "The Stigmatized Image of the 'Crack Head': A Sociocultural Exploration of a Barrier to Cocaine Smoking Among a Cohort of Youth in New York City." *Deviant Behavior* 20: 153–81.

General Accounting Office (GAO). 1990. *Methadone Maintenance: Some Treatment Programs Are Not Effective; Greater Federal Oversight Needed.* Washington, D.C.: G.A.O.

Goldstein, Paul J., Douglas S. Lipton, Edward Preble, Ira Sobel, Tom Miller, William Abbott, William Paige, and Frank Soto. 1984. "The Marketing of Street Heroin in New York City." *Journal of Drug Issues* 14, no. 3: 553–66.

Golub, Andrew L., Farrukh Hakeem, and Bruce D. Johnson. 1996. *Monitoring the Decline in the Crack Epidemic with Data from the Drug Use Forecasting Program: Final Report to National Institute of Justice.* New York: John Jay College of Criminal Justice.

Golub, Andrew L., and Bruce D. Johnson. 1994a. "Cohort Differences in Drug Use

Pathways to Crack Among Current Crack Abusers in New York City." *Criminal Justice and Behavior* 21, no. 4: 403–22.

―――. 1994b. "A Recent Decline in Cocaine Use Among Youthful Arrestees in Manhattan, 1987–1993." *American Journal of Public Health* 84, no. 8: 1250–54.

―――. 1996. "The Crack Epidemic: Empirical Findings Support a Hypothesized Diffusion of Innovation Process." *Socio-Economic Planning Sciences* 30, no. 3: 221–31.

―――. 1997. "Crack's Decline: Some Surprises Across U.S. Cities." *Research in Brief.* Washington, D.C.: National Institute of Justice.

―――. 1998. "Substance Use Progression and Hard Drug Abuse in Inner-City New York." In *Stages and Pathways of Involvement in Drug Use: Examining the Gateway Hypothesis.* Edited by Denise Kandel. New York: Cambridge University Press.

―――. 1999. "Cohort Changes in Illegal Drug Use Among Arrestees in Manhattan: From the Heroin Injection Generation to the Blunted Generation." *Substance Use and Misuse* 34, no. 13: 1733–63.

―――. 2001. *The Rise of Marijuana as the Drug of Choice Among Youthful Arrestees.* Washington, D.C.: National Institute of Justice.

Golub, Andrew, Bruce D. Johnson, and Tracy Durrah. 1999. *Drug Use Among Arrestees in the Five Boroughs of New York City (Third Quarter 1998 to First Quarter 1999).* Occasional Report no. 2 from the ADAM-New York City Program.

Gray, Mike. 1998. *Drug Crazy: How We Got into This Mess and How We Can Get Out.* New York: Random House.

Hamid, Ansley. 1992. "The Developmental Cycle of a Drug Epidemic: The Cocaine Smoking Epidemic of 1981–1991." *Journal of Psychoactive Drugs* 24: 337–48.

Hamid, Ansley, R. Curtis, K. McCoy, J. McGuire, A. Conde, W. Bushell, R. Lindenmayer, K. Brimberg, S. Maia, S. Abdur-Rashid, and J. Settembrino. 1997. "The Heroin Epidemic in New York City: Current Status and Prognoses." *Journal of Psychoactive Drugs* 29: 375–91.

Hartman, Donna, and Andrew Golub. 1999. "The Social Construction of the Crack Epidemic in the Print Media." *Journal of Psychoactive Drugs* 31, no. 4.

Hunt, G. Halsey, and Maurice E. Odoroff. 1962. "Follow-up Study of Narcotic Drug Addicts After Hospitalization." *Public Health Reports* 77, no. 1: 41–54.

Hunt, Leon. 1973. *Heroin Epidemics: A Quantitative Study of Current Empirical Data.* Washington, D.C.: Drug Abuse Council.

Hunt, Leon G., and Carl D. Chambers. 1976. *The Heroin Epidemics: A Study of Heroin Use in the U.S. Part 2, 1965–75.* Holliswood, N.Y.: Spectrum.

Iiyama, Patti, Nishi Sutsuko, and Bruce D. Johnson. 1976. *Drug Use and Abuse Among U. S. Minorities: An Annotated Bibliography.* New York: Praeger.

Inciardi, James A., and Lana D. Harrison, eds. 1998. *Heroin in the Age of Crack Cocaine.* Beverly Hills, Calif.: Sage.

Jaffe, Jerome. 2002. "One Bite of the Apple: Establishing the Special Action Office for Drug Abuse Prevention." In this volume, chap. 4.

Johnson, Bruce, Terry Williams, Kojo Dei, and Harry Sanabria. 1990. "Drug Abuse and the Inner City: Impact on Hard Drug Users and the Community." In *Drugs and Crime*. Edited by Michael Tonry and James Q. Wilson. Crime and Justice Series, vol. 13. Chicago: University of Chicago Press.

Johnson, Bruce D. 1973. *Marihuana Users and Drug Subcultures*. New York: Wiley.

———. 1975a. "Righteousness Before Revenue: The Moral Crusade Against the Indo-Chinese Opium Trade." *Journal of Drug Issues* 5, no. 4: 304–26.

———. 1975b. "Understanding British Addiction Statistics." *Bulletin on Narcotics* 27, no. 1: 49–66.

———. 1975c. "Interpreting Official British Statistics on Addiction." *International Journal of Addictions* 10, no. 4: 557–88.

———. 1976. "The Social Functioning of Opiate Maintenance Clinics in London and New York City." *British Journal of Addictions* 71: 175–82.

———. 1980. "Towards a Theory of Drug Subcultures." In *Theories on Drug Abuse: Selected Contemporary Perspectives*. Research Monograph 30. Edited by Dan Letteri et al. Rockville, Md.: NIDA.

———. 1984. "Empirical Patterns of Heroin Consumption Among Selected Street Heroin Users. " In *Social and Medical Aspects of Drug Abuse*. Edited by George Serban. Jamaica, N.Y.: Spectrum.

Johnson, Bruce D., Eloise Dunlap, and associates. 1998. *Natural History of Crack Distribution/Abuse: Final Report to National Institute on Drug Abuse*. New York: National Development and Research Institutes.

Johnson, Bruce D., Eloise Dunlap, and Lisa Maher. 1998. "Nurturing for Careers in Drug Abuse and Crime: Conduct Norms for Children and Juveniles in Crack-Abusing Households." *Substance Use and Misuse* 33, no. 7: 1515–50.

Johnson, Bruce D., Paul J. Goldstein, Edward Preble, James Schmeidler, Douglas S. Lipton, Barry Spunt, and Thomas Miller. 1985. *Taking Care of Business: The Economics of Crime by Heroin Abusers*. Lexington, Mass. Lexington Books.

Johnson, Bruce D., Andrew L. Golub, and Eloise Dunlap. 2000. "The Rise and Decline of Drugs, Drug Markets, and Violence in New York City." In *The Crime Drop in America*. Edited by Alfred Blumstein and Joel Wallman. Cambridge: Cambridge University Press.

Johnson, Bruce D., Andrew L. Golub, and Jeffrey Fagan. 1995. "Careers in Crack, Drug Use, Drug Distribution, and Nondrug Criminality." *Crime and Delinquency* 41, no. 3: 275–95.

Johnson, Bruce D., and John Muffler. 1997. "Sociocultural." In *Substance Abuse*. Edited by Joyce Lowinson et al. Baltimore: Williams and Wilkins.

Johnson, Bruce D., Mangai Natarajan, Eloise Dunlap, and Elsayed Elmoghazy. 1994. "Crack Abusers and Noncrack Abusers: Profiles of Drug Use, Drug Sales, and Nondrug Criminality." *Journal of Drug Issues* 24, no. 1–2: 117–41.

Johnson, Bruce D., George Thomas, and Andrew L. Golub. 1998. "Heroin Use Among Manhattan Arrestees from the Heroin and Crack Eras." In *Heroin in the Age of Crack Cocaine*. Edited by James Inciardi and Lana Harrison. Beverly Hills, Calif.: Sage.

Johnston, Lloyd. 1991. "Towards a Theory of Drug Epidemics." In *Persuasive*

Communication and Drug Abuse Prevention. Edited by L. Donohew, H. Sypher, and W. Bukoski. Hillsdale, N.J.: Erlbaum.

Joseph, Herman, and Phil Appel. 1985. "Alcoholism and Methadone Treatment: Consequences for the Patient and Program." *American Journal of Drug and Alcohol Abuse* 11: 37–53.

Joseph, Herman, Vincent P. Dole, and James Schmeidler. 1983. "Predicting Post-Treatment Narcotic Use Among Patients Terminating from Methadone Maintenance." *Advances in Alcohol and Substance Abuse* 2, no. 1: 57–68.

Kelling, George L., and Catherine M. Coles. 1996. *Fixing Broken Windows: Restoring Order and Reducing Crime in Our Communities*. New York: Free Press.

King, Rufus. 1972. *The Drug Hang-up: America's Fifty-Year Folly*. 2d ed. Springfield, Ill.: Charles C. Thomas.

Krogh, Egil, Jr. 2002. "Heroin Politics and Policy Under President Nixon." Chapter 3 in this volume.

Lipton, Douglas S., Gregory Falkin, and Harry K. Wexler. 1991. "Correctional Drug Treatment in the United States." *Professional Counseling* 6: 39–44, 57.

Lipton, Douglas S., and Bruce D. Johnson. 1998. "Smack, Crack, Score: Two Decades of NIDA-Funded Drugs and Crime Research at NDRI, 1974–1994." *Substance Use and Misuse* 33, no. 9: 1779–1815.

Lowinson, Joyce, J. Thomas Payte, Edwin Walsitz, Herman Joseph, Ira J. Marion, and Vincent Dole. 1997. "Methadone Maintenance." In *Substance Abuse*. Edited by Joyce Lowinson et al. Baltimore: Williams and Wilkins.

Lowinson, Joyce, Pedro Ruiz, Robert Millman, and John Langrod, eds. 1997. *Substance Abuse: A Comprehensive Textbook*. 3d ed. Baltimore: Williams and Wilkins. (Hereafter, Lowinson et al. 1997.)

Malcolm X and Alex Haley. 1966. *The Autobiography of Malcolm X*. New York: Ballantine.

Massing, Michael. 1998. *The Fix*. New York: Simon and Schuster.

Milby, J. B. 1988. "Methadone Maintenance to Abstinence. How Many Make It?" *Journal of Nervous and Mental Disease* 176, no. 7: 409–22.

Morgan, H. Wayne. 1981. *Drugs in America: A Social History*. Syracuse, N.Y.: Syracuse University Press.

Musto, David. 1973. *The American Disease: Origins of Narcotic Control*. New Haven, Conn.: Yale University Press.

———. 1974. "Early History of Heroin Addiction in the United States." In *Addiction*. Edited by Peter Bourne. New York: Academic Press.

———. 1991. "Opium, Cocaine and Marijuana in American History." *Scientific American* (July): 40–47.

———. 1993. "The Rise and Fall of Epidemics: Learning from History." In *Drugs, Alcohol, and Tobacco: Making the Science and Policy Connections*. Edited by Griffith Edwards, John Strang, and Jerome H. Jaffe. New York: Oxford University Press.

———. 1994. "Faith in the Legal Control of Drugs: Then and Now." *New York State Bar Journal* 66 (May/June): 14–17.

———. 2002. "Introduction." In this volume.

Musto, David, and M. R. Ramos. 1981. "Notes on American Medical History: A Follow-up Study of the New Haven Morphine Maintenance Clinic of 1920." *New England Journal of Medicine* 304: 1071–77.

National Advisory Commission on Civil Disorders. 1968. *U.S. Riot Commission Report*. New York: Bantam Books.

National Institute of Justice. 1997. *Drug Use Forecasting 1996: Annual Report on Adult and Juvenile Arrestees*. Washington, D.C.: National Institute of Justice.

National Institute of Justice. 1998. *1997 Annual Report on Adult and Juvenile Arrestees*. Washington, D.C.: National Institute of Justice.

National Institute of Justice. 1999. *1998 Annual Report on Drug Use Among Adult and Juvenile Arrestees*. Washington, D.C.: National Institute of Justice.

New York City Bar Association. 1976. *Effects of the 1973 Drug Laws on New York State Courts*. Rockville, Md.: National Institute of Justice.

Nurco, David. 1998. "A Long-Term Program of Research on Drug Use and Crime." *Substance Use and Misuse* 33, no. 9: 1817–37.

O'Donnell, John A. 1969. *Narcotic Addicts in Kentucky*. Washington, D.C.: Department of Health, Education, and Welfare, National Institute of Mental Health.

O'Donnell, John A., Harwin L. Voss, Richard R. Clayton, Gerald T. Slatin, and Robin G. Room. 1976. *Young Men and Drugs: A Nation-wide Survey*. Rockville, Md.: National Institute on Drug Abuse.

Office of Applied Studies. 1999. *Year-end 1997 Preliminary Emergency Department Data from the Drug Abuse Warning Network*. Washington, D.C.: Substance Abuse and Mental Health Services Administration.

Preble, Edward. 1975. Personal communication regarding history of heroin in East Harlem.

Preble, Edward, and John Casey. 1969. "Taking Care of Business: The Heroin User's Life on the Streets." *International Journal of Addictions* 4 (March): 1–24.

Preble, Edward, and Bruce D. Johnson. 1978. *The Ethnography of Two White Ethnic Groups*. New York: Narcotic and Drug Research.

Preble, Edward, and Thomas Miller. 1977. "Methadone, Wine, and Welfare." In *The Ethnography of Drugs and Crime*. Edited by Robert Weppner. Beverly Hills, Calif.: Sage.

Reinarman, Craig, and Harry G. Levine. 1997. *Crack in America: Demon Drugs and Social Justice*. Berkeley: University of California Press.

Reuter, Peter, and Robert MacCoun. 2002. "Heroin Maintenance: Is a U.S. Experiment Needed?" Chapter 10 in this volume.

Rittenhouse, Joan D., ed. 1977. *The Epidemiology of Heroin and Other Narcotics*. Rockville, Md.: National Institute on Drug Abuse.

Rogers, Everett M. 1995. *Diffusion of Innovations*. 4th ed. New York: Free Press.

Schafer, D. Paul. 1998. *Culture: Beacon of the Future*. Westport, Conn.: Praeger.

Schneider, Eric C. 1999. *Vampires, Dragons, and Egyptian Kings: Youth Gangs in Postwar New York*. Princeton, N.J.: Princeton University Press.

Shilts, Randy. 1987. *And the Band Played On: Politics, People, and the AIDS Epidemic*. New York: Penguin.

Stoneburner, R. L., D. Des Jarlais, D. Benezra, L. Gorelkin, J. L. Sotheran, S. R.

Friedman, S. Schultz, M. Marmor, D. Mildvan, and R. Maslansky. 1988. "A Larger Spectrum of Severe HIV-1-Related Disease in Intravenous Drug Users in New York City." *Science* 242: 916–19.

Substance Abuse and Mental Health Services Administration (SAMHSA). 1999. *Summary of Findings from the 1998 National Household Survey on Drug Abuse.* DHHS Publication no. SMA99-3328. Rockville, Md.: SAMHSA.

Terry, Charles, and Mildred Pellens. 1928. *The Opium Problem.* New York: Bureau of Social Research.

Thomas, Piri. 1967. *Down These Mean Streets.* New York: Knopf.

Waldorf, Dan. 1971. "Compulsory Treatment in New York City's Candy-Coated Jails." *Drug Forum* (September).

———. 1973. *Careers in Dope.* Englewood Cliffs, N.J.: Prentice-Hall.

———. 1998. "Misadventures in the Drug Trade." *Substance Use and Misuse* 33, no. 9: 1957–91.

Waldorf, Dan, and Patrick Biernacki. 1981. "Natural Recovery from Heroin Addiction: Some Preliminary Findings." *Journal of Drug Issues* 11, no. 1.

Waldorf, Dan, Martin Orlick, and Craig Reinarman. 1974. *The Shreveport, Louisiana, Morphine Maintenance Clinic, 1919–1923.* Washington, D.C.: Drug Abuse Council.

White, William L. 2002. "Trick or Treat? A Century of American Responses to Heroin Addiction." Chapter 7 in this volume.

Wilson, Orlando W. 1963. *Police Administration.* 2d ed. New York: McGraw-Hill.

Wilson, William J. 1996. *When Work Disappears: The World of the New Urban Poor.* New York: Random House.

Wish, Eric D., Elizabeth Brady, and Mary Cuadrado. 1984. "Drug Use and Crime of Arrestees in Manhattan." Paper presented at 47th annual meeting of Committee on Problems of Drug Dependence, St. Louis.

Wish, Eric D., and Bruce D. Johnson. 1986. "The Impact of Substance Abuse on Criminal Careers." In *Criminal Careers and "Career Criminals."* Edited by Alfred Blumstein, Jacqueline Cohen, Jeffrey A. Roth, and Christy A. Visher. *Vol. 2, Panel on Research on Criminal Careers.* Washington, D.C.: National Research Council. Pp. 52–88.

Wolfgang, Marvin E., and Franco Ferracuti. 1967. *The Subculture of Violence.* London: Tavistock.

Part IV

Treatment Options

8

Trick or Treat?
A Century of American
Responses to Heroin Addiction

William L. White

When Congress passed the 1972 Drug Abuse Treatment Act, it forged a federal-state-local partnership that called for shared responsibility in the design, implementation, operation, and evaluation of community-based, multimodality narcotic addiction treatment programs across the United States. American approaches to the treatment of narcotic addiction evolved over the course of a century from the first professionalization of addiction treatment in the 1870s to the rise of these modern multimodality treatment systems in the late 1960s and early 1970s. Changing treatment technologies fall into five overlapping periods that collectively laid the foundation for the current system for treating heroin addicts in America. Several themes are particularly significant to this story of national policy, including the vacillating views on the etiology and nature of heroin addiction, the competing claims of institutional ownership of the heroin problem, the shift in the goal of treatment from personal recovery to containment of social costs, and the enduring ambivalence (if not outright hostility) toward narcotic maintenance.

THE PRE-HEROIN WORLD OF ADDICTION
TREATMENT, 1830–98

America's earliest narcotic addiction problems were iatrogenic in nature. They were spawned by the isolation of morphine and codeine, the introduction of the hypodermic syringe, the widespread distribution of opiate drugs by physicians, and the aggressive marketing of opiate-laced medicines (such as Dr. McMunn's Elixar of Opium and Mrs. Winslow's Soothing Syrup) by a multimillion-dollar patent medicine industry whose sales grew from $3.5 million in 1859 to $74.5 million in 1903. Narcotic addiction arose in a nineteenth-century America that had few nonnarcotic alternatives for the management of acute and chronic disease or trauma (Musto 1985; Courtwright 1982; Young 1961).

Nineteenth-century addicts, like many of their twentieth-century counterparts, were likely to find themselves in generalist systems of care that lacked any special knowledge of, or specialized approaches to, the treatment of narcotic addiction. Many addicts sought help from private physicians—sometimes the same physicians who had been the source of their introduction to opiates. Others sought discreet detoxification in such nonspecialty institutions as water-cure establishments or private rest homes. Still others found themselves coerced into private hospitals or legally committed by family members to state insane asylums.

New Institutions and Medicines

Growing concerns about alcoholism, narcotic addiction, and addiction to nonnarcotic drugs, such as cocaine and bromides, during the second half of the nineteenth century—as well as the perception that existing institutions were not adequately responding to these problems—prompted the founding of the first specialized addiction treatment facilities in America. Five overlapping institutional or medicinal approaches developed in the emerging field of addiction treatment, reflecting differences in ideology, affiliation, or patient base. *Inebriate homes*, like the Washingtonian Homes of Boston and Chicago, usually were sponsored by religious or temperance organizations that viewed addiction recovery as a process of moral reformation. More medically oriented *inebriate asylums*, such as the New York State Inebriate Asylum, arose under private or state auspices. The inebriate homes and asylums were linked organizationally with the founding of the American Association for the Study and Cure of Inebriety in 1870 and through the association's central organ, the *Journal of Inebriety*. These institutions embraced all addictive disorders within the umbrella concept of inebriety, which was viewed as an inherited or acquired "disease" that could be cured with appropriate treatment (*Proceedings, 1870–1875* 1981).

Private proprietary institutes and sanataria also were established. Some of them—for instance, the Keeley Institutes, Neal Institutes, and Gatlin Institutes—operated as for-profit addiction cure franchises with branches all over the country. Such institutes catered to affluent narcotic addicts, including many physicians and others from the professional classes. Most clients of inebriate homes, inebriate asylums, and proprietary institutes were there for the treatment of alcoholism, but these institutions did admit narcotic addicts. There were also *private facilities specializing in the treatment of narcotic addiction.* These included the DeQuincey Home, operated by Dr. H. H. Kane, and the Brooklyn Home for Habitués, operated by Dr. J. B. Mattison. Finally, there were *bottled home cures* for narcotic addiction, promoted by the same patent-medicine industry that spewed opiate-laced home remedies across the land. These medicinal specifics that claimed to cure narcotic addiction—products with such names as Denarco, Opacura, and Antidote—almost all contained high dosages of morphine and provided little more than disguised drug maintenance (Adams 1906).

Treatment Methodologies

Nineteenth-century treatment methods for narcotic addiction focused almost exclusively on withdrawal and brief physical convalescence. There were three general approaches: (1) abrupt withdrawal over twenty-four to thirty-six hours, (2) rapid withdrawal over four to ten days, and (3) gradual withdrawal over a period of weeks or months. A wide variety of pharmacological adjuncts were utilized to facilitate withdrawal: narcotic substitutes, such as codeine; nonnarcotic substitutes, such as cannabis or cocaine; tonics, including whiskey or strychnine; sedatives, such as chloral hydrate and paraldehyde; purgatives, which were thought to speed the elimination of narcotic poisons; and belladonna derivatives, such as hyoscine (scopolamine) and atropine, which brought on intoxication, delirium, and forgetfulness that tended to prevent the addict from fleeing during the withdrawal process.

Agents used to reduce narcotic craving included aversive drugs, like tartar emetic, and plants such as *Avena sativa* (White 1998). The choice of some of these pharmacological treatments is surprising by today's standards. American physicians as early as 1880 were prescribing cocaine (by the pound) as a treatment for morphine addiction and reporting as a testament to cocaine's effectiveness that their patients were requesting additional quantities of cocaine and that they had completely lost their appetite for morphine (Bentley 1880). Withdrawal and postwithdrawal convalescence were also aided by such treatment adjuncts as hydrotherapy, electrical stimulation, massage, specialized diets, and special exercise regimens.

Autobiographical accounts by nineteenth-century narcotic addicts describe such treatments as excruciating and uniformly ineffective (see Day 1868; Cobbe 1895; Eubank 1903). Relapse rates were exceptionally high but were shrouded from the public behind the advertised cure rates of addiction treatment institutes—claims that usually exceeded 95 percent and were based on either a patient's status at discharge or the percentage of patients who did not apply for readmission.

This makeshift system of narcotic addiction treatment collapsed in the first two decades of the twentieth century. A decline in morphine addiction produced by new prescription laws and improved physician education, public exposés of unethical and fraudulent treatment practices, economic depressions, and state (and then national) alcohol prohibition laws all worked to decrease demand for addiction treatment institutions and to reduce the public and philanthropic financial resources that had supported such institutions (White 1998).

Had the system survived, however, it would have been ill-suited to the demands of the new times, for early twentieth-century heroin addicts could not have been more different from their nineteenth-century morphine-addicted counterparts. Heroin addicts were more likely to be male rather than female, and young, as opposed to middle-aged; to live in the urban centers of the North, rather than in the rural South; to be children of new European immigrants rather than of the native-born; and to use narcotics for pleasure rather than for relief of pain.

The new addicts were viewed as incorrigible rather than sick. Whereas the addiction of the nineteenth-century medical (morphine) addict was classified as "involuntary" and the user portrayed as an innocent victim of an unduly stigmatized disease, the behavior of the new twentieth-century criminal (heroin) addict was classified as "voluntary." The addiction of this new population was considered, if not simply a vice, then a "self-inflicted disease" (Flowers and Bonner 1923; Simon 1924).

There were other differences. Morphine addicts typically had sustained their addiction in secrecy and isolation from one another, but heroin addicts took part in a pattern of "freemasonry and cooperation" within an elaborately organized illicit drug subculture (Bailey 1916). Most significant, the new heroin addicts generally had neither the social standing nor the financial resources to gain access to the remnants of what was in essence a private treatment system (Terry and Pellens 1928). As heroin sniffing and then heroin injecting spread in the early twentieth century, what was needed was not a refinement of nineteenth-century treatment methods but a newly configured approach to treatment, based on an understanding of heroin and the characteristics of those who were being drawn to it.

THE CLINIC AND COMMUNITY HOSPITAL PERIOD, 1894–1924

Three public policy milestones marked the shift in the treatment of narcotic addiction in the United States during the second decade of the twentieth century: (1) the passage of the Harrison Tax Act in 1914, (2) the interpretation of the act's strictures concerning physicians in the 1919 *Webb v. United States* Supreme Court decision, and (3) the failure of the France Bill to pass Congress in 1919. The first two events produced the de facto criminalization of the status of addiction in the United States.

The Narcotics Division of the Treasury Department took the position that since acceptable cures were available, addicts should not be maintained on narcotics. Physicians who did maintain addicts on their usual and customary doses were considered under the Harrison Act, as confirmed in the *Webb v. United States* decision, not to be practicing in "good faith," and were subject to arrest. More than twenty-five thousand physicians were indicted under the Harrison Act between 1919 and 1935, and twenty-five hundred of this number were sentenced to prison (Williams 1935, 1938). The France Bill, introduced in 1919, provided a unique window of opportunity to alter the early course of American narcotics control policy. The bill would have provided federal funds for local communities to establish addiction treatment programs and to utilize the services of the U.S. Public Health Service hospitals as a backup for these community-based services. The failure of this measure even to come to a vote placed the responsibility for the care of addicts squarely on the shoulders of local communities.

Many communities responded by establishing narcotics clinics to care for addicts. These clinics maintained incurable and infirm addicts on stable doses of narcotics while encouraging more able-bodied addicts to undergo detoxification via gradual outpatient withdrawal or rapid withdrawal in local hospitals. The goals of the clinics were twofold: (1) to provide consistent medical management of narcotic addicts and (2) to suppress the illicit drug traffic by preventing drug peddlers from preying upon confirmed addicts.

The clinics varied greatly in their level of success. Some, like those operated by the State Board of Public Health in Shreveport, Louisiana, and by the New Haven, Connecticut, Police Department, were highly regarded, while others, such as the Worth Street Clinic in New York City, were castigated for their disorganization and ineffectiveness. Neither the Worth Street Clinic nor Riverside Hospital, where addicts enrolled in the Worth Street Clinic were encouraged to complete their detoxification, produced any notable cures among the thousands of addicts they admitted (Graham-Mulhall 1921). The clinic approach, christened "ambulatory treatment," came under bitter attack from law enforcement authorities and from the national medical establishment (Federal Bureau of Narcotics 1955; Council on Mental Health, AMA 1966). During the early 1920s, all of the clinics closed under threat of indictment. America's brief experiment with morphine and heroin maintenance had been declared a failure by administrative fiat of the Narcotics Division of the Treasury Department.

The fledgling specialty of addiction medicine was all but obliterated between 1914 and 1924. Physicians who continued to treat narcotic addicts in their local communities did so at great peril to their professional reputations and licenses–risks that for most were just too great. It would be more than fifty years before significant numbers of physicians again involved themselves in the ongoing care of heroin addicts. With the closing of the last clinic, responsibility for the care of incurable addicts was removed from physicians and turned over to criminal syndicates.

THE VACUUM, 1924–35

Isolated voices of protest against this demedicalization and criminalization of addiction didn't alter the reality that, between 1924 and 1935, there were almost no resources available for the treatment of narcotic addicts. While affluent, middle-aged addicts sought discreet detoxification in a new generation of postasylum private hospitals—such as the Charles B. Towns Hospital for Drug and Alcoholic Addictions in New York City—a growing number of young heroin addicts were more likely to undergo withdrawal in a jail cell than in a hospital bed. When state-supported inebriate asylums closed, states did loosen commitment laws to allow for the admission of addicts into state psychiatric hospitals, but few of these facilities provided any specialized approach to the treatment of addiction. Almost the only exception to this rule was the California State Narcotics Hospital at Spadra, which provided institutional treatment for addicts from 1928 to 1941 (Joyce 1929).

Physicians within private and community hospitals continued to focus on the problem of narcotic withdrawal. Withdrawal regimes going by such names as the Towns-Lambert Treatment, the Pettey Method, the Nellens and Masse Method, and Narcosan vied for prominence as a means of quickly detoxifying addicts. But there was growing agreement that most of these methods produced few enduring cures. The vision of a medicinal specific that could cure narcotic addiction gave way to pessimism in the late 1920s (Musto 1973).

The shift from viewing addicts as diseased to viewing them as depraved marked a new era of coercive and invasive methods of suppressing and managing addiction. Addicts denied access to hospitals entered the criminal justice system in ever-increasing numbers. A eugenics movement that attributed America's social problems to bad breeding successfully lobbied for inclusion of addicts in state mandatory sterilization laws. Inebriate commitment laws were expanded to provide for the involuntary commitment of narcotic addicts to state insane asylums. As heroin use became increasingly associated with young male criminals, it was proposed that addicts be indefinitely quarantined in inebriate colonies, so that addiction could be prevented from spreading to the larger community.

It is perhaps not surprising in this context that perceptions of the causes of addiction shifted from discussions of the addict's diseased cells to arguments about his or her psychopathic character (compare Crothers 1902; Bishop 1912; or Pettey 1913 with Kolb 1925). Perhaps this growing climate of contempt for the addict can help us understand the introduction of brutally invasive cures during the opening decades of the twentieth century. There were the "serum therapies," which involved raising blisters on the addict's abdomen and thighs, withdrawing the fluid from the blisters, and then reinjecting it into the addict over several days of withdrawal (Reddish 1931). There were the "blood therapies," which, similarly, consisted of withdrawing blood from the addict and then reinjecting it over the course of withdrawal. There were sodium thiocyanate-based withdrawal therapies that could induce psychoses lasting as long as two months (Bancroft and Rutzler 1931). But even these treatments paled next to the "bromide sleep treatments" that continued to be recommended as a withdrawal strategy in spite of earlier reports of a 20 percent death rate (Church 1900).

THE NARCOTIC FARM ERA, 1935–65

Calls for the creation of specialized hospitals for the treatment of narcotic addicts increased during the 1920s from such influential persons as Dr. Lawrence Kolb of the U.S. Public Health Service. These calls became more strident by 1928, when more than two-thirds of federal inmates were identified as addicts. Overcrowding produced by the growing numbers of addicts entering federal prisons and the lack of any systematic approach to their care led to congressional passage of the Porter Act in 1929. This measure called for the creation of two "narcotics farms" to be operated by the U.S. Public Health Service. The first of these farm-hospital-prison amalgams opened in Lexington, Kentucky, in 1935 and the second opened in Fort Worth, Texas, in 1938. These institutions treated both addicted prisoners and addicts who volunteered for treatment. All addicts coming from east of the Mississippi River were treated at Lexington; those from west of the Mississippi River were treated at Fort Worth. Lexington could accommodate fourteen hundred inmates at a time, and Fort Worth, a thousand.

Between 1935 and the late 1950s, the Lexington and Fort Worth facilities constituted the primary source of addiction treatment in the United States. Treatment at the U.S. Public Health hospitals was divided into three phases: withdrawal, convalescence, and rehabilitation. The evolving character of the illicit drug culture is revealed in the changing profile of the addicts admitted to Lexington and Fort Worth. The self-medicating aged and infirm addict continued to give way to the young addict; morphine continued to give way to heroin as the addict's drug of choice; and nonwhite admissions increased from 12 percent in 1936 to 56 percent in 1966 (Cuskey et al. 1972).

Treatment at Lexington and Fort Worth was administered by interdisciplinary teams of physicians, psychiatrists, nurses, social workers, chaplains, and recreational therapists. Following drug-aided withdrawal, inmates were moved to wards where they spent most of their time working in such institutional industries as farming, landscaping, and construction—labor for which they were reimbursed with cigarettes. The length of stay was variable and problematic. Involuntary patients stayed too long (because of the length of their sentences), while voluntary patients often decided to leave before staff felt they were stable enough to avoid relapse. Evaluations of discharged patients from Lexington and Fort Worth consistently concluded that 90–95 percent of those discharged returned to the use of narcotics (Maddux 1978). The Lexington and Fort Worth facilities were sustained until their function began to be taken over by the rise of local community-based addiction treatment. The Fort Worth facility was closed in 1971 and the Lexington facility in 1974. With these closures, the responsibility for operating addiction treatment facilities officially shifted from the federal government back to the states and local communities.

During the federal farm period, those addicts not treated at Lexington and Fort Worth could, with sufficient resources, still be treated by private physicians, be cared for in private settings such as the Towns Hospital, or become subjects in a growing number of local treatment experiments that began in the 1950s. Most addicts, however, were likely to find themselves in jail or a psychiatric institution. Whether at a private psychiatric hospital such as the Menninger Foundation in Topeka, Kansas, or one of many large and overcrowded state psychiatric hospitals, addicts were subjected to whatever was currently in vogue in psychiatric care. Private hospitals were heavily influenced by psychoanalytic thinking that portrayed addiction as a sexually derived character disturbance in the same category as kleptomania, Don Juanism, and gambling. Treatment, this argument followed, should take the form of several months of rest in a sanatorium and individual psychoanalysis (Knight and Prout 1951).

While the use of methadone as a highly effective aid to withdrawal began at the U.S. Public Health hospitals as early as 1948, withdrawal treatments outside these settings remained quite primitive. The range of experimental treatments that addicts were subjected to in psychiatric institutions, prison hospitals, and community care settings is astounding. The serum (blister) cures continued to be practiced in the 1930s in settings like the Colorado State Penitentiary. The 1940s and 1950s witnessed the use of electroconvulsive therapy and insulin shock therapy as an aid to withdrawal; "hibernation therapy" (withdrawal aided by sodium pentothal narcosis); the use of apomorphine (induced nausea) and succinyl choline (induced fear of suffocation) to create an aversion to narcotics; the experimental use of psychosurgery (the prefrontal lobotomy) as an addiction treatment; the use of LSD as an adjunct in psychotherapy with addicts; the use of antipsychotic drugs (phenothiazines) in narcotic withdrawal; and the use of methamphetamine as a medically prescribed substitute for heroin (Kleber and Riordan 1982).

It should not be surprising that, in response to such invasive and ineffective treatments, the first American mutual aid society for narcotic addicts was founded in this period. The roots of Narcotics Anonymous (N.A.) can be traced to "Addicts Anonymous" meetings at the U.S. Public Health Hospital in Lexington in 1947, which were organized by Houston S., a member of Alcoholics Anonymous (A.A.). N.A.'s program of mutual support mirrored A.A.'s Twelve Steps and Twelve Traditions. N.A. struggled to survive in the 1940s and 1950s but eventually grew to a membership of more than 250,000 active members in the 1990s (Stone 1997). Many treatment programs would eventually establish linkages with N.A. similar to those they had earlier developed with A.A.

THE RISE OF COMMUNITY-BASED TREATMENT

Two interrelated events set the stage for the rise of local experiments in the treatment of narcotic addiction. The first was a dramatic rise in juvenile narcotic addiction in the early 1950s, and the second was the passage of laws in 1952 (the Boggs Act) and 1956 (the Narcotic Control Act) that dramatically increased penalties for possession and sale of narcotics—including the first penalty options for life imprisonment and execution. These draconian measures spurred many groups to reexamine narcotics policy. Studies that portrayed addiction as a product of poverty and social deprivation, joint committee reports of the American Bar Association and the American Medical Association, and recommendations of the Presidential Advisory Commission on Narcotics and Drug Abuse all provided momentum for increased experimentation with more effective responses to the problem of drug addiction.

Additional momentum came from a 1962 Supreme Court decision (*Robinson v. California*) declaring that narcotic addiction was a disease and that addicts were "proper subjects for medical treatment." A few states experimented with state-operated addiction treatment hospitals, including Blue Hills Hospital in Connecticut and Avon Park in Florida. Local experiments spawned in this climate included a variety of church-sponsored addiction ministries, particularly in Chicago and New York City. Addict wards were established in some community hospitals (Manhattan General Hospital, for instance) and a special institution, Riverside Hospital, was opened in New York City specifically for the treatment of juvenile narcotic addicts.

Communities across the United States needed a means of responding to rising rates of addiction. What was required to fill this need were replicable models of addiction treatment. Two approaches to the treatment of heroin addiction emerged that met this replicability criteria: the therapeutic community (TC) and methadone maintenance (MM).

TCs for the treatment of drug addiction were born in 1958 when Charles Dederich began an experimental mutual aid community called Synanon. While Synanon would not sustain its focus on addict rehabilitation, its early years set the model for TCs all over the United States. This model called for an addict's sustained (one-to-two-year) enmeshment in a confrontational but also caring community of recovering addicts—a community that provided an authoritarian surrogate family in which the addict was pushed to regress, was resocialized, and then was given progressively greater responsibility and contact with the outside community. TCs defined the etiology of addiction characterologically and defined recovery as a process of emotional maturation. By 1975 there were more than five hundred TCs in the United States modeled after Synanon (Yablonsky 1965; Mitchell et al. 1980).

MM was pioneered in 1964 by Drs. Marie Nyswander and Vincent Dole, who conceptualized heroin addiction as a metabolic disease and introduced the daily oral administration of methadone as a means of stabilizing the addict's disordered metabolism, so that full rehabilitation could be possible. With appropriate doses of methadone, addicts discovered a zone of stable functioning that prevented acute intoxication on the one hand and narcotic withdrawal on the other. Following positive evaluations of the pilot sites, MM programs were established in urban areas across the United States. By 1973 more than eighty thousand heroin addicts were being maintained on methadone in licensed treatment programs scattered across the American urban landscape (Dole and Nyswander 1968; Dole 1997).

Other methods of treating heroin addiction in the 1960s and 1970s included renewed experiments with civil commitment programs, the use of narcotic antagonists as a treatment adjunct, alternative maintenance agents, new nonopiate withdrawal medications (for example, clonidine), new withdrawal adjuncts (for example, acupuncture), and the introduction of new treatment monitoring tools in the form of drug testing and aggressive case management. All of these approaches were integrated within a growing network of federal- and state-funded treatment programs. In Connecticut, Illinois, and New York, methadone detoxification and maintenance (both residential and outpatient), residential therapeutic communities, outpatient drug-free programs, and a growing number of new special-populations programs began to be integrated within multimodality treatment systems. By 1975 there were more than eighteen hundred local drug treatment programs in the country supported by a newly forged federal and state partnership. The modern era of addiction treatment had begun.

THEMES IN HEROIN TREATMENT

I would offer the following closing observations regarding the evolution of heroin addiction treatment in America.

Trends

The story of heroin addiction in America is a story of changing heroin potency, changing methods of heroin administration, changing motivations for heroin use, changing characteristics of heroin users, and the emergence and changing nature of the illicit drug culture in America. Views of heroin addiction and its treatment at any point in time must be defined within the context of these elements.

Problem Perception

Perceptions of the etiology of heroin addiction have placed the locus of vulnerability for addiction within the biology of the addict (disease conceptualizations), the moral or emotional architecture of the addict (characterological explanations), and the social environment of the addict (sociological explanations). Early treatments reflected single- pathway models that posited a singular causative agent and a singularly narrow approach to treatment. Later multiple-pathway (ecological) models have suggested varied and interacting etiological influences, have identified multiple clinical sub-populations, and have stressed the need for highly individualized approaches to treatment. These latter models emphasize the importance of understanding initiating and sustaining (consolidating) factors in heroin addiction and the interaction of biological, psychosocial, and spiritual dimensions to addiction and recovery.

Role of the Physician

Supervision of the heroin addict was removed from physicians in the early twentieth century and turned over to criminal syndicates and the criminal justice system. The major story of the last half of the twentieth century is the rebirth of addiction medicine and the rising responsibility of the physician in the treatment of heroin addiction. Only time will tell whether this involvement is sustainable.

Treatment Environment

Cyclical and coexisting trends of isolation and integration mark the treatment of heroin addiction in the United States. During periods in which the addict is demonized and addiction is portrayed as contagious, addicts are socially extruded (quarantined) in the name of treatment. The sequestration of incurable addicts was effected in a most unusual way in the United States. By criminalizing addiction, the American prison system, without acknowledgment, absorbed the functions set forth in early proposals for the establishment of addict colonies. During periods of greater social stability and less fear, efforts have been made to localize the treatment of addicts within non-institutional models of care.

Treatment Specifics

Since the mid-1800s, narcotic addiction specialists have sought a specific—a pharmacological intervention that could restore the addict's cells and psyche to their preaddiction state. To date, that search has failed. It is unlikely that any drug, by itself, will ever be capable of severing the addict's relationship with heroin and the life-transforming subculture in which its use is imbedded.

Treatment Methods

The major achievement in the treatment of heroin addiction in the twentieth century is the recognition that narcotic withdrawal does not in and of itself constitute treatment. All our advancements have grown out of this shift from the preoccupation with the mechanics of withdrawal to the more difficult issues of managing drug craving and chronic drug-seeking behavior.

New Treatments

New breakthroughs announced in the treatment of heroin addiction are notoriously unreliable. Hope-inspiring claims nearly always break down in the face of controlled studies and cumulative clinical experience.

Treatment Replication

The most positively evaluated treatment innovations often have been corrupted during the course of widespread replication. Such replications are marked by a loss of the core technology as well as by a shift in focus from one of personal recovery for the addict to social control of the addict. Such problems were encountered in the replication of both therapeutic communities and methadone maintenance. Dr. Vincent Dole, the codeveloper of methadone maintenance, memorably remarked, "The stupidity of thinking that just giving methadone will solve a complicated social problem seems to me beyond comprehension" (Courtwright et al. 1989).

Treatment Intensity

What late twentieth-century models of narcotic addiction—dating from the original designs of the therapeutic community and methadone mainte-nance—held in common was the belief that treatment needed to be charac-terized by high intensity and long duration. That is, there was a belief that positive treatment outcomes were related to treatment dose—both qualita-tively and quantitatively. This premise is being challenged by a system of behavioral health care that is using an acute care model of low-intensity, brief interventions in both the public and private sector. This broader contextual shift could pose the greatest threat to the future of treatment for heroin ad-diction by shifting the focus from sustained recovery maintenance to serial episodes of acute detoxification.

Drug Maintenance

The consistently positive evaluation, by statistical measures, of narcotic maintenance, in spite of widespread infidelity to the original model, has done very little to alter most Americans' continued negative feelings (ranging from ambivalence to open hostility) about this modality.

Addict Vulnerability

Addicts (and their families) are exceptionally vulnerable to exploitation. The social demonization of the addict, the political manipulation of the re-sulting fear of addicts, capitalization on the issue of addiction for personal and bureaucratic gain, and the presence of fraudulent cures are enduring themes in the history of heroin addiction in the twentieth century.

Treatment Harm

The term "iatrogenic addiction" has been used to denote addiction spawned by the use of heroin as a medical treatment—a phenomenon, as David Courtwright has documented in this volume, that was not a major problem. But there is another, more relevant use for the term "iatrogenic" (physician-caused) harm in this arena, and that is regarding the injury that has been done to addicts under the auspices of care. When one considers a history of addiction "treatments" that include agonizing withdrawal regimes, multiyear legal institutionalizations, psychosurgery, electroconvulsive therapy, serum therapy, and the administration of a wide spectrum of toxic and aversive drugs, it is clear that harm done in the name of good is an enduring thread within the history of addiction treatment in America.

Lack of Voice

The voices of American narcotic addicts, in contrast to those of addicts in some European countries or of American alcoholics, have rarely been heard on questions of social policy or treatment. There has been no indigenous "modern narcotic addiction movement" mirroring the achievements of the "modern alcoholism movement." No grassroots consumer movement has yet impacted narcotic addiction treatment in America.

Mutual Aid

A major factor in alcoholism recovery in America has been the rise of A.A. and other mutual aid societies and the local linkages established between these groups and alcoholism treatment agencies. In contrast, linkages between agencies treating heroin addiction and N.A. have not reached the same level, either quantitatively or qualitatively. N.A. remains one of the most potentially beneficial but underutilized resources in long-term recovery from heroin addiction.

Addiction as a Chronic Disease

An emerging model of narcotic addiction treatment views such addiction for a significant percentage of addicts as a chronic disease characterized by periods of remission and relapse. Such a view suggests that addicts may need different types of treatment and support services at different points in their addiction/recovery careers. In terms of treatment matching, this model suggests not just that different treatments need to be carefully matched to particular addicts but also that the same addict may require different treatments at different points in time. This model further posits the thesis that treatment episodes need to be evaluated not in terms of their event effect (that is, the short-term outcome of a single treatment episode) but in terms of their cumulative effect on the addict's addiction and recovery careers.

Natural Resources

There has been a growing recognition through studies of what has been variously christened "maturing out," "spontaneous remission," and "natural recovery" that there are sources of resiliency within the addict and within the addict's natural environment that can aid addiction recovery (Winick 1962; Biernacki 1986). The most successful treatments of the future will find ways to align themselves with these natural forces.

Problem Ownership

Heroin addiction was one of the intractable problems of the twentieth century. The ownership of such problems is inherently unstable (Room 1978). Americans' ambivalence about a drug that promises not only relief from pain but also pleasure and escape; our disregard and contempt for people associated with this drug's use; and our fear that those close to us are, or could be, within this drug's reach have kept ownership of this problem forever shifting across the boundaries of religion, law, and medicine. In which arena, and where within each arena, an addict was likely to be involved during any decade of the twentieth century has been influenced primarily by issues of age, gender, race, social class, and region.

Vulnerability of Treatment Systems

Systems of addiction treatment—think of, for instance, the broad nineteenth-century network of inebriate homes and asylums, the early twentieth-century maintenance clinics, and the mid-twentieth-century federal narcotics hospitals—are prone to collapse in the face of any or all of the following conditions: highly publicized ethical abuses, economic depressions that erode their financial viability, a public image as a place where the rich or the bad are coddled and protected from the consequences of their behavior, a shift from medical to criminal models of viewing addiction (usually during a period of fear of social disorder), failure to develop a credible treatment technology, and the failure to address problems of leadership development and succession (White 1998).

In this chapter I have reviewed the history of addiction from the pre-heroin world through the rise of a community-based treatment system during the early 1970s. The birth, operation, achievements, and shortcomings of the federal-state-local addiction treatment partnership of the late twentieth century are described in later chapters of this book.

REFERENCES

Adams, S. 1906. "The Scavengers." *Collier's Weekly*, September 22, pp. 112–13. (Reprint series).

Bailey, Pearce. 1916. "The Heroin Habit." *New Republic* 6 (April 22): 314–16.

Bancroft, W., and J. Rutzler. 1931. "Reversible Coagulation in Living Tissue." *Proceedings of the National Academy of Science* 71: 138.

Bentley, W. 1880. "Erthroxylon Coca in the Opium and Alcohol Habits." *Detroit Therapeutic Gazette* 1: 253–54.

Biernacki, P. 1986. *Pathways from Heroin Addiction: Recovery Without Treatment.* Philadelphia: Temple University Press.

Bishop, E. 1912. "Morphinism and Its Treatment." JAMA 58 (May 18): 1499–1504.

Brooklyn Home for Habitués. 1891. *Quarterly Journal of Inebriety* (July): 271–72.

Church, A. 1900. "The Treatment of the Opium Habit by the Bromide Method." *New York Medical Journal* 71: 904.

Cobbe, W. 1895. *Doctor Judas: A Portrayal of the Opium Habit.* Chicago: S. C. Griggs.

Council on Mental Health, American Medical Association. 1966. "Review of the Operation of the Narcotic 'Clinics' Between 1919–1923." In *Narcotic Addiction.* Edited by J. O'Donnell and J. Ball. New York: Harper & Row. Pp. 180–87.

Courtwright, D. 1982. *Dark Paradise: Opiate Addiction in America Before 1940.* Cambridge, Mass.: Harvard University Press.

Courtwright, D., H. Joseph, and D. Des Jarlais. 1989. *Addicts Who Survived: An Oral History of Narcotics Use in America.* Knoxville: University of Tennessee Press.

Crothers, T. D. 1902. *Morphinism and Narcomanias from Other Drugs.* Philadelphia: W. B. Saunders.

Cuskey, W., T. Premkumar, and L. Sigel. 1972. "Survey of Opiate Addiction Among Females in the United States Between 1859 and 1970." *Public Health Review* 1: 5–39.

Day, H. B. 1868. *The Opium Habit, with Suggestions as to the Remedy.* New York: Harper & Brothers.

Dole, Vincent. 1997. "What is 'Methadone Maintenance Treatment'?" *Journal of Maintenance in the Addictions* 1, no. 1: 7–8.

Dole, V., and M. Nyswander. 1968. "Successful Treatment of 750 Criminal Addicts." JAMA 206: 2710–11.

Eubank, R. 1903. *Twenty Years in Hell; or, the Life, Experience, Trials and Tribulations of a Morphine Fiend.* Kansas City: Revelation.

Federal Bureau of Narcotics. 1955. *Narcotic Clinics in the United States.* Washington D.C.: U.S. Government Printing Office, Pp. 1–23.

Flowers, M., and H. Bonner. 1923. *The Menace of Morphine, Heroin and Cocaine.* Pasadena, Calif.: Narcotic Education Association.

Graham-Mulhall, S. 1921. "Experiences in Narcotic Drug Control in the State of New York." *New York Medical Journal* 113: 106–11.

Joyce, T. 1929. "California State Narcotic Hospital." *California and Western Medicine* 31 (September): 190–92.

Kleber, H., and C. Riordan. 1982. "The Treatment of Narcotic Withdrawal: A Historical Review." *Journal of Clinical Psychiatry* 43, no. 6: 30–34.

Knight, R., and C. Prout. 1951. "A Study of Results in Hospital Treatment of Drug Addictions." *American Journal of Psychiatry* 108: 303–8.

Kolb, L. 1925. "Types and Characteristics of Drug Addicts." *Mental Hygiene* 9: 300–13.

Kolb, L., and C. Himmelsbach. 1938. "Clinical Studies of Drug Addiction: A Critical Review of the Withdrawal Treatment with Method of Evaluating Abstinence Syndromes." *American Journal of Psychiatry* 94: 759–97.

Lowry, J. 1956. "The Hospital Treatment of the Narcotic Addict." *Federal Probation* 15: 20.

Maddux, J. 1978. "History of the Hospital Treatment Program: 1935–1974." In *Drug Addiction and the US Public Health Service*. Edited by W. Martin and H. Isbell. DHEW Pub. no. ADM-77-434. Pp. 217–50.

Mitchell, D., C. Mitchell, and R. Ofshe. 1980. *The Light on Synanon*. New York: Seaview.

Musto, D. 1973. *The American Disease: Origins of Narcotic Control*. New Haven, Conn.: Yale University Press.

—————. 1985. "Iatrogenic Addiction: The Problem, Its Definition and History." *Bulletin of the New York Academy of Medicine* 2d ser., 61 (October): 694–705.

Pettey, George. 1913. *Narcotic Drug Diseases and Allied Ailments*. Philadelphia: F. A. Davis.

Proceedings 1870–1875, American Association for the Cure of Inebriates. 1981. New York: Arno.

Reddish, W. 1931. "The Treatment of Morphine Addiction by Blister Fluid Injection." *Kentucky Medical Journal* 29: 504.

Room, R. 1978. "Governing Images of Alcohol and Drug Problems: The Structure, Sources, and Sequels of Conceptualizations of Intractable Problems." Ph.D. diss., University of California, Berkeley.

Senay, E., and P. Renault. 1971. "Treatment Methods for Heroin Addicts: A Review." *Journal of Psychoactive Drugs* 3, no. 2: 47–54.

Simon, C. 1924. "Survey of the Narcotic Problem." *JAMA* 82: 675–79.

Stone, B. 1997. *My Years with Narcotics Anonymous*. Joplin, Mo.: Hulon Pendleton.

Terry, C. E., and M. Pellens. 1928. *The Opium Problem*. Montclair, N.J.: Patterson Smith.

Vogel, V. 1948. "Treatment of the Narcotic Addict by the United States Public Health Service." *Federal Probation* (June): 45–50.

Waldorf, D., and P. Biernacki. 1979. "The Natural Recovery from Heroin Addiction: A Review of the Incidence Literature." *Journal of Drug Issues*. 9: 281–89.

White, W. 1998. *Slaying the Dragon: The History of Addiction Treatment and Recovery in America*. Bloomington, Ill.: Chestnut Health Systems.

Williams, H. 1935. *Drugs Against Men*. New York: Robert M. McBride.

Williams, H. 1938. *Drug Addicts Are Human Beings*. Washington, D.C.: Shaw.

Winick, C. 1962. "Maturing Out of Narcotic Addiction." *Bulletin on Narcotics* 14, no. 5 (January-March).

Yablonsky, L. 1965. *Synanon: The Tunnel Back*. Baltimore: Penguin.

Young, J. 1961. *The Toadstool Millionaires: A Social History of Patent Medicines in America Before Federal Regulation*. Princeton, N.J.: Princeton University Press.

9

Methadone:
The Drug, the Treatment, the Controversy

Herbert D. Kleber

The current methadone controversy is the most recent round in a policy struggle that has been going on since 1964, when the first program began. An appropriate quotation with which to begin a discussion of this rocky history might be the old line "No good deed goes unpunished." Many consider methadone treatment one of the really good deeds, if not great deeds, in the history of the treatment of addiction, yet it clearly is also one of the most assailed.

Methadone was discovered by the Germans during World War II, when they had opiate shortages because of problems with sea routes. After the war it was taken over by Lilly Pharmaceutical and named Dolophine. Some of the anti-methadone groups have claimed the name came from Adolph Hitler and that it is used to weaken the African American community. Actually, Dolophine was named from the Latin *dolor* (pain). Supporters believe that its use can relieve addicts' pain and free them from enslavement to heroin.

After World War II, research on methadone was carried out at the Addiction Research Center in Lexington, Kentucky. The papers from those early days are fascinating. Researchers had little to go on in terms of appropriate dosage. In some studies they put addicts on doses as high as 350 to 400 mg, and then abruptly stopped. The patients would withdraw "cold turkey," and the staff would carefully chart what the patients went through As one of them said, "Man, this stuff never lets you go." Three weeks later, four weeks later, they would still be suffering withdrawal symptoms.

As more became known about the drug, however, unwanted effects were reduced and the benefits became clear. It began to replace morphine or codeine, the drugs in main use in the late 1940s and early 1950s, as the preferred agent to detoxify individuals from heroin. In 1964 Vincent Dole, an internist, and Marie Nyswander, a psychiatrist, developed the use of methadone as a maintenance drug. Dole had started from the point of view that heroin addiction was really a metabolic disease. Using an insulin model, he had looked for a maintenance drug. Nyswander had written a book based on her experience in treating addicted jazz musicians and the frustrations and difficulties that ensued. She was searching for a medication that would improve outcome. The two, working at Rockefeller University, were trying different maintenance agents; when they got to methadone, they found that their patients behaved very differently. They began to make their beds; they began to talk about wanting to go to work. From that humble beginning, the idea of methadone as a maintenance drug took shape.

There are many key players in this history. Jerry Jaffe, Mary Jean Kreek, Frances Gearing, and Joyce Lowinson have all played major roles in the spread of methadone since the mid-1960s. The controversy about methadone then and now is captured in an anecdote from 1966. At that time I was at the U.S. Public Health Service hospital in Lexington, Kentucky, running one of the addiction treatment units. A program called Daytop Village had just started in New York, and I invited the director to give a talk to the patients at Lexington—although the word "patients" may not be quite accurate: Lexington was a prison. Two-thirds of the thousand residents were serving sentences of from one to ten years. The remaining one-third were voluntary admittees, who signed in because at that time it was the only place to get treatment for narcotic addiction in the United States east of the Mississippi, as its counterpart prison hospital in Fort Worth, Texas, was for west of the Mississippi. The Daytop director talked about therapeutic communities, and, during a question-and-answer period, one of the patients asked about methadone, which they had just heard about. The response was a classic remark: "I think methadone maintenance is a great idea: we should give money to bank robbers, women to rapists, and methadone to addicts."

That was 1966. Five years later the speaker went on to head a methadone program. So life treats us in funny ways. But it is one of my favorite anecdotes because it captures the feeling that a lot of people still have about methadone maintenance—that it constitutes immoral pandering to criminals rather than a scientific treatment of a disease.

In 1968 methadone began to spread out of New York. Jerry Jaffe began his program in Chicago, Bill Weiland started in Philadelphia, and I began in New Haven. All of these programs were supported by NIMH grants. In New Haven we set up a model multimodality treatment program with central intake.

Methadone was just one of the modalities we were using. We also had a therapeutic community, an adolescent program, and narcotic antagonists. In those
days, cyclazocine was the antagonist of choice. Also during that era, we
learned you didn't need to admit everyone as an inpatient to start, as they
did at Rockefeller. Bill Weiland began outpatient induction. We started
patients on a day program, which became a fixture in New Haven for many
years, to deal with the fact that many of our addicts basically needed re-
socialization. Anyone who was not working was required to come in 9:00–
4:30 five days a week. During that time they had intensive group therapy,
individual therapy, and help with vocational and educational issues. I credit
the success of our methadone program in large part to those initial six weeks,
which helped to break the code of the streets and to get people involved in
wanting to lead not simply a life on methadone, but a whole different life.

As methadone was spreading, so was the controversy. There was continued opposition from therapeutic communities. I was at a number of meetings in those days where, if it was predominantly a TC audience and someone
got up to speak about methadone, he would get booed; if it was primarily a
methadone audience and someone got up to speak about TCs, *he* would get
booed.

There was also a lot of opposition from the black community, some of
whom described methadone maintenance as genocidal—an attempt by the
white establishment to control young black males by keeping them permanently addicted. I remember vividly one episode during the Black Panther
trial in New Haven. Some of the members of that group came to me and said,
"If you don't close your methadone program, we're going to burn it down."
Their rationale was not that it was not successful, but that it was *too* successful: it helped addicts quit heroin but did not deal with the conditions in the
ghetto that they believed *produced* addiction—such as racism, unemployment,
and poverty. They viewed it as putting a sort of Band-Aid on the ghetto, an
attempt to avoid the total revolution they believed would soon happen.

I believe the thinking was somewhat similar to what the Communists did
in the 1930s, trying to kill off the labor unions. The feeling was that labor
unions would give the workers half a loaf, and if you did that, they would
not rise up and overthrow the whole economic system. These feelings about
methadone from some members of minority communities have never totally
gone away, although at times they are more prominent than at others. In any
event, our clinics neither closed down nor burned down, but instead grew
and prospered, because of the help patients were getting.

In retrospect, the 1970s was the golden era of methadone. Bob DuPont
in Washington, D.C., showed that you could rapidly develop a large system
and bring a great number of the addicts in the city into quality treatment.
The federal government encouraged the spread of methadone maintenance

via Bud Krogh, Jerry Jaffe, and SAODAP. By 1973 there were approximately four hundred methadone programs throughout the United States. The National Institute on Drug Abuse (NIDA) was founded, and it was used initially not simply to do research but also to spread methadone programs.

During that same era, there were a number of studies on methadone safety. There were a lot of myths on the street then about methadone: it got into your bones, it ate away your teeth, it destroyed your vision. In systematically looking at those systems where the street rumors had it that methadone was dangerous—including the kidneys, the eyes, the musculoskeletal system, and the heart—our group at Yale in five-year studies, and Mary Jean Kreek in New York in eight-year studies, found no evidence of any damage due to protracted methadone use. We concluded that addicts could be on methadone for at least five to eight years without adverse physical effects.

Another question began to emerge: Should people be on methadone for life, or, if you rehabilitate them, can they be detoxed and remain abstinent? Dole and Nyswander advocated very strongly, if not the universal lifetime model, then at least keeping patients on methadone for many years—some, perhaps, for their whole life. They believed that being on heroin for many years changed the addict's brain and changed his metabolism, probably permanently.

Our program in New Haven took a different direction. We believed that if you could rehabilitate addicts, you would be able to get them off methadone, especially if you could solve the withdrawal problem. We spent a lot of energy looking at a variety of ways of doing detoxification. From that interest, we demonstrated that clonidine, on the market for hypertension, could markedly decrease withdrawal symptoms, and that combining clonidine and naltrexone could yield a rapid opioid detox with even better results. These methods increased the likelihood that people who had been successfully rehabilitated could get off methadone. While these techniques improved on existing approaches, we still do not have good enough methods by which to end reliance on methadone, and I believe that is one of the major problems. We're not going to know how long people need to be on methadone until we have a much better way of detoxifying them. Buprenorphine is one of the drugs that may help in the future to resolve the controversy as to what percentage of recovering addicts need to remain on methadone versus what percentage can successfully detox from it.

I have a favorite anecdote about the detox controversy. Dole and Nyswander came up to visit our program and give a seminar. One of our counselors, a former methadone patient who had been clean for about six months, asked a lot of pointed questions about the theory that methadone had to be taken for life. When the seminar was over and we went out for dinner, Marie and Vince said, "Tell us about that guy who was asking all the questions. Has he been on methadone and is now withdrawing?" I replied, "Yes, he's been clean for six months." They then said, "Ah, we thought so. It's that irritability due to the protracted methadone withdrawal that really got him to ask all those questions." Perhaps that was the case, perhaps not, but it reveals the strong feelings of even such wonderful researchers as these two. Parenthetically, the counselor was able to stay off heroin, and methadone, for decades.

While there were other problems in the 1970s, including concerns about methadone overdose among children and nonaddicts who might become exposed to the drug and about methadone diversion, in many ways it was the golden era, a time when, for the most part, methadone was respected and seen as an important part of the treatment system for addicts.

In the 1980s there was a backlash. Early in that decade, the federal block grant replaced direct NIDA grants as a way of funding drug programs. Each state received a certain amount of money that could be used for methadone or for other kinds of treatment, and you began to see a discontinuation of methadone in a number of places. The best study of this natural experiment was the one in Bakersfield County, headed by Bill McLaughlin. What they found when they looked at the patients who were detoxed of necessity, because the clinics were closed, was that, while some stayed clean and some found treatment in other counties, many did not fall into either of those categories. Among this latter group, there were an increased number of deaths and of return to heroin addiction, and an increased amount of criminal activity. Unfortunately, this study did not carry much weight. One of the things I learned in my days in government is that, much as we are reluctant to admit it, science does not drive policy. It may push it a bit—policymakers say they would like to know the science—but, at the end of the day, that is not how they make their decisions.

During the Reagan years, some of the White House drug policy advisers were quite anti-methadone. I think of Carlton Turner, for example. That viewpoint peaked in 1988 with the White House Conference for a Drug Free America, which was vehemently anti-methadone. They demonized it, as well as NIDA, which they viewed as being "soft on drugs," and they called for a congressional investigation of that agency. This time was probably the lowest point methadone reached, in terms of national policy.

Also during the 1980s, however, evidence was accumulating about the relationship of methadone programs and HIV status. Studies showed that individuals on methadone had a much lower incidence of conversion to HIV-positive status. In England the harm reduction movement was taking hold, driven by the concern over AIDS. The English made a conscious decision in the mid-to-late 1980s that preventing AIDS was more important than dealing optimally with drug abuse, and that, therefore, the main focus of their drug program should be reducing the spread of the HIV virus rather than re-habilitating addicts. The philosophy that flowed from this decision was that no matter how badly a patient is doing on methadone—no matter how much cocaine he is doing, how much alcohol he is drinking, whether he is involved in criminal behavior, and so forth—you keep him on methadone, because if you throw him off, instead of using drugs once a day or once every other day, he will go back to using three or four times a day, and increase the likelihood of HIV conversion.

This attitude took hold in the United States as well, although some of us continued to take the position that the best way to prevent HIV was to offer good-quality treatment with high rather than low expectations. Also during the 1980s, we had the rise of private, for-profit methadone programs. One of the things I am proud of is that during my years in Connecticut I fought to keep for-profit methadone out of the state. Unfortunately, after I left Connecticut in 1989, that Horatio-at-the-bridge position was lost. In other states it was lost a lot earlier. In California, for example, by 1990, 90 percent of their two hundred methadone clinics were privately owned. The major source of funds was patient fees. Between 1980 and 1990, there was an 80 percent increase nationally in reliance on patient fees as the primary source of funding for methadone programs. Along with the rise of the for-profit programs came a curtailment in services.

In the mid-1970s the "slot cost" for a methadone slot was roughly $1700 a year. In 1990 the Institute of Medicine committee on treatment effectiveness that David Courtwright and I, among others, served on showed that from 1976 to about 1986, funding for methadone had increased by only about 9 percent, from $1700 a slot to $1850 a slot, while costs went up by at least 35 to 40 percent during those years of high inflation. This disparity eroded the ability of clinics to provide services, and the spread of for-profit programs had a similar effect: if you provided fewer services, you could make more money.

Clinics developed where you would go in and a drawer like the one on an ATM would come out. You'd put in your credit card, your cash, or your Medicaid card, the drawer would be pulled back, and then it would be pushed forward again, and you'd get your card back, with your dose of methadone. On the wall there typically would be a sign that said, "If you want counseling, please ask one of the staff." Unfortunately, from being the exception in the 1970s, that kind of program has proliferated; and it has had, I believe, a negative impact on public perception. If the methadone patients are basically being maintained but not treated, if the public sees that these patients continue to use cocaine and continue to engage in criminal behavior, they are going to ask, Why should we be paying for this? Why should we permit it?

In the 1990s, when I was Deputy Director for Demand Reduction under Bill Bennett at the Office of National Drug Control Policy, we tried to reverse this movement and to increase respect again for methadone treatment. We put out a White Paper which said very clearly that methadone maintenance was both a legitimate and an important part of the spectrum of drug abuse treatment. We doubled the federal funding for treatment, so that services would be expanded and improved. Unfortunately, the resulting increase in funding accomplished less than we had hoped, because, as we found out later, while we were putting money in the front door via the block grant, the states were pulling out their contributions to program funding through the back door. I tried to get Congress to pass a law that would have made that more difficult, but they were not interested. They said that the Department of Health and Human Services (HHS) already had the power to do that if they wanted to. Unfortunately, HHS was not interested in such a law, nor even in using the power they already had to prevent this supplanting of funds.

The issue of "interim methadone" or "low-threshold methadone" was raised during this period in relation both to the AIDS issue and to the fact that it was very hard to expand methadone treatment. During much of the 1990s, we had about 120,000 methadone slots for somewhere between 750,000 and 850,000 heroin addicts. That's less than one slot for every six potential patients, so there was a push by many people concerned with drug treatment to adopt the so-called Hong Kong model with ten thousand people on methadone and eleven social workers doing therapy. Similarly, in the Netherlands, the dose of methadone was kept low so that patients could continue to use heroin if they wished, and addicts could drop in and out of the program.

I don't like these models. The definitive study, I believe, was Tom McLellan's beautifully designed study, published in JAMA in 1984, which randomly assigned addicts to one of three groups: methadone only, methadone as usual (methadone with one counseling session a week), or enhanced methadone (not just drug counselors but also psychologists, psychiatrists, and medical help). At the end of three months, they found that the first group was doing so badly that, for ethical reasons, they felt they had to take two-thirds of them out of the methadone-only protocol and move them into one of the other two types of programs. The enhanced methadone group had markedly lower levels of heroin and cocaine use, needle sharing, and unemployment. Within a few months, the new patients in the groups with counseling were doing just as well as the people who had been there from the beginning. So it clearly was not the patients who accounted for the different results; it was the program. If you have low expectations and minimal services for your patients, they respond appropriately. If you have higher expectations and better services, they respond to that, too.

At the same time these studies were going on, the Dutch were beginning to find out that their methadone policy was flawed. The Amsterdam Health Department published a paper showing that its low-threshold, low-dose methadone approach did not reduce HIV risk. That led to some rethinking of their position. They retained the low-threshold requirement but adopted higher dose levels.

Increasingly, however, states curtailed the length of time patients were allowed to be on methadone maintenance. Oklahoma limited addicts to one year on methadone over a lifetime. Office-based dispensing also aroused disagreements. The central question was Should people continue indefinitely to have to come to a methadone clinic to obtain the drug, or should they be able to get methadone in a doctor's office? Some people argue for allowing physicians to dispense the drug at the beginning of treatment; others want it only after stabilization and improvement, as one way of increasing the number of methadone slots. I have trouble with the former. I don't have trouble with the latter.

At the same time as these controversies were taking place, the scientific community was confirming the efficacy of methadone treatment. An NIH consensus statement in 1997 asserted the value of methadone. In 1998 General McCaffrey pronounced probably the strongest support I have heard from any director of the Office of National Drug Control Policy: "Methadone is very important to our strategy."

Support of the harm reduction philosophy in the 1990s, however, contributed to decreasing services in methadone programs. At the second national methadone consumers meeting in October 1998, for instance, the argument was the following: "Since methadone doesn't treat cocaine, and that's not why we're in methadone treatment, use of cocaine should never be considered an indication for termination from methadone. Patients should get lower or higher doses as they choose, and they should have the right to have low doses so they can continue to use heroin without the harder override caused by a high dose of methadone."

As is probably evident, I do not agree with much of that harm reduction position. One of the things I've learned in running a methadone program is that drug use is contagious. If you have a program with vigorous support and high expectations, your patients live up to that: you create a program with a relatively low use of other drugs compared to the average clinic. Since many methadone patients want to use other drugs—they are, after all, individuals who enjoy the effects of drugs, whether they be heroin, cocaine, alcohol, or marijuana—once a program permits some patients to use without consequences, the amount of illicit drug use that goes on in the program markedly increases. My experience has been that the more relaxed programs are, and the more tolerant of drug use, the more they have both drug use and other illicit activities. No one should be surprised by this outcome.

In the summer of 1998, New York City launched its welfare-to-work program. Only about 20 percent of methadone patients were legally employed, and Mayor Giuliani concluded that methadone programs needed to do a better job of getting their patients to work. Unexpectedly, he announced a plan to eliminate methadone maintenance in the city. Of the approximately thirty-six thousand methadone slots in New York City at the time, only about two thousand were controlled by the city. The rest were controlled by New York State, which indicated no interest in cutting methadone. Nonetheless, the plan was highly controversial and generated heated debate.

In the rush to defend methadone and methadone patients that ensued, advocates lost sight of some unpleasant realities. According to the city Health and Hospitals Corporation, for instance, the employment rate in methadone programs in the city ranged, at that time, from a low of 15 percent in the Bronx to a high of 25 to 30 percent in Staten Island and Queens. The reasons are not mysterious. Addicts in many of these programs are on Medicaid, which pays the program over $100 per week. If the patient goes to work and earns perhaps $15,000–$20,000 a year, he may be able to pay the program only $10–$20 per week. If the program accepts that, they are losing up to a hundred dollars. So it is neither in their interest to encourage the patient to go to work, nor in the patient's interest to do so.

I hear from colleagues that the employment rate is a lot higher than 15 to 30 percent, but often it is off the books. Neither the programs nor the patients have an interest in making employment public knowledge when it might result in patients losing welfare and Medicaid—and, perhaps, access to methadone. While this may not be as much an issue in programs less dependent on reimbursement, it certainly is in other methadone programs. A reasonable solution might be to permit people to continue in treatment for a period after they leave welfare—through interim funding, for example.

How was the mayor's statement received? There was no outcry from the majority of people in New York, including the leaders of the black community, many of whom had complained about the mayor in other circumstances. The black community was ambivalent about methadone at best; many of its leaders were hostile toward methadone treatment. Thus they were not unhappy when the mayor attacked methadone clinics. The policy also played very well in conservative upstate New York and other places in the country. While various prestigious scientific organizations, such as the American Psychiatric Association, defended methadone, they were joined by neither key political leaders nor a substantial number of voters.

This should worry treatment specialists more than what a single city official does. Giuliani's order to eliminate methadone and substitute abstinence programs was rescinded after six months. In fact, the mayor decided to add $5 million in new funding to the city-run methadone programs, to improve staffing levels and overall quality of service. I was asked to work with the New York City programs to help achieve this, and spent a year doing so. The programs are now called Narcotic Addiction Treatment Programs. Eventually they will offer both maintenance and abstinence programs. Some patients will be on methadone maintenance, others on buprenorphine or naltrexone. I see this as a future direction for existing methadone programs in general.

Over the long run, programs that lack political support have trouble competing for resources. Methadone supporters should acknowledge reasonable concerns, such as getting patients to work and preventing Medicaid abuses. High levels of cocaine abuse should be a signal for needed change, not defended as inevitable. On the wall of the therapeutic community that is part of the New Haven program I directed, there is a plaque that says, "You are neither the giant of your dreams nor the pygmy of your fears." Methadone is not the panacea for our heroin problem; it is not the perfect treatment for heroin addiction, but neither is it the demon that some people would like to make it. The truth lies somewhere in the middle.

Note: This overview of medical practitioners' experience with methadone is adapted from an after-dinner talk, thus, the informal tone and absence of scientific citations.

10

Heroin Maintenance: Is a U.S. Experiment Needed?

Peter Reuter and Robert MacCoun

Methadone maintenance repeatedly has been shown to be the most effective available treatment for a large fraction of heroin addicts.[1] Given that fewer than half of entrants, on average, stay in a methadone program in the United States for as much as one year, and that most continue to use illegal drugs even during that time, the disappointing implication is that the United States has a weak armamentarium for dealing with the problem of heroin addiction.[2] Heroin addiction appears to be very long-lasting, with many addicts from the 1970s still, in the 1990s, dependent on the drug and involved in high-risk health and crime behaviors.[3] It is hardly surprising that there is a continuing interest in finding alternatives that would bring some surcease to both the user and society.

Heroin maintenance has long been one of those alternatives. Maintenance clinics were part of the initial response to the Harrison Act and famously were shut down (a process of some years during the 1920s) after a close-fought legal battle was resolved in favor of the hawkish-on-drugs Treasury Department. Some historians have pointed approvingly to the Shreveport and New Orleans clinics; others have focused on the mismanaged New York clinic to suggest that they did little good and much damage.[4] But the idea of providing heroin to addicts as a humane harm-reduction measure has reappeared from time to time in the U.S. drug policy debate, and, largely because of European developments, it is moderately prominent once again at the turn of the century.

So far, attention has centered on the possibility of conducting a U.S. demonstration or trial; immediate implementation of heroin maintenance on a large scale is not being discussed. Yet even the notion of a trial has been highly controversial. It is not merely drug hawks, unsympathetic to the plight of dependent drug users, who believe this notion is both morally and pragmatically flawed; even researchers long involved in drug treatment and clearly very concerned about addicts' well-being have been antagonistic. The prospects are bleak indeed.

We believe that a reasonable case can be made for a U.S. trial. The recent Swiss trials, for all the methodological weaknesses of their evaluation, provide evidence of feasibility and a prima facie case for effectiveness. The downside risks of a trial in the United States seem slight and the potential benefits, substantial. However, the Swiss evidence does not provide an adequate basis to make a decision about the desirability of heroin maintenance as a policy option in the United States. Extrapolating from foreign experiences is difficult in any field of social policy, and it is easy to identify characteristics of programs, patients, and context that render the Swiss trials weak evidence for projecting what would happen here. Hence, the need for U.S.-based trials.

That is not to say that the critics are without a case. Some issues can be resolved without a field trial. The first is that heroin maintenance raises fundamental normative concerns; for some, these trump any possible public health gains. Swiss pragmatism and American idealism may derive different conclusions from the same set of results about the effects of providing a highly addictive drug to those who already crave it. Later in this chapter, we will identify some ethical issues, generally resolving them in favor of allowing for the possibility of adopting heroin maintenance if it proves to be substantially better than other modalities for a significant fraction of America's six hundred thousand to eight hundred thousand heroin addicts. There are also important political arguments that have been raised as objections to a heroin maintenance trial; we will describe those as having more power. Finally, we will consider programmatic arguments, identifying the limits of small-scale experiments to answer fundamental questions.

Before embarking on this discussion, in the next section we provide a brief review of Britain's long experience with heroin maintenance, highlighting the fact that British doctors have made very little use of their right to provide the drug since the mid-1970s. The following section summarizes the implementation of the Swiss field trials and describes the reaction to it in Switzerland, the United States, and elsewhere. That is followed by a discussion of normative and political issues. Finally, we identify the potential for a heroin trial in the United States.

THE BRITISH EXPERIENCE

In a 1926 report, the blue-ribbon Rolleston Committee concluded that "morphine and heroin addiction . . . must be regarded as a manifestation of disease and not as a mere form of vicious indulgence." Thus, if repeated attempts to withdraw a patient from cocaine or heroin were unsuccessful, "the indefinitely prolonged administration of morphine and heroin [might] be necessary [for] those [patients] who are capable of leading a useful and normal life so long as they take a certain quantity, usually small, of their drug of addiction, but not otherwise" (as quoted in Stears 1997, 123). This led the British government to adopt, or at least to formalize, a system in which physicians could prescribe heroin to addicted patients for maintenance purposes (Judson 1974). With a small addict population, composed chiefly of iatrogenically addicted opiate users (numbering in the hundreds), the system muddled along for four decades with few problems (Spear 1994).

The system was not very controversial throughout most of that period. When the Tory government in 1955 considered banning heroin completely, in response to international pressures rather than because of any domestic complaints about the system, the British medical establishment fought back effectively, and the government eventually abandoned the effort. However, the incident seemed to say more about the power of the medical establishment and its dedication to physician autonomy than about the success of heroin maintenance (Judson 1974, 29–34).

Then, in the early 1960s, a very small number of physicians began to prescribe irresponsibly, and a few heroin users began using the drug purely for recreational purposes, recruiting others like themselves (Spear 1994). The result was a sharp proportionate increase in heroin addiction in the mid-1960s, although it still left the nation with a very small heroin problem; there were only about fifteen hundred known addicts in Britain in 1967 (Johnson 1975). In response to the increase, the Dangerous Drugs Act of 1967 greatly curtailed access to heroin maintenance, limiting long-term prescriptions to a small number of specially licensed drug-treatment specialists.[5] General practitioners were not unhappy to be rid of the responsibility for dealing with a population of long-term patients who were difficult to manage and showed only modest improvements in health over the course of treatment.

Addicts could now be maintained over the long term only in clinics. At the same time, oral methadone became available as a substitute pharmacotherapy. British specialists proved as enthusiastic about this alternative as did their U.S. counterparts, though initially they did not expect long-term maintenance to be the norm, and injectable methadone played a significant role. The fraction of maintained addicts receiving heroin fell rapidly. By 1975, just 4 percent of maintained opiate addicts were receiving only heroin; another

8 percent were receiving both methadone and heroin (Johnson 1977). That reluctance to prescribe heroin remains the case today; less than 1 percent of those being maintained on an opiate receive heroin (Stears 1997). The strong and continued antipathy of British addiction specialists to the provision of heroin is a curious and troubling phenomenon for those who advocate its use.[6]

British research on the efficacy of heroin maintenance is quite limited. One classic study (Hartnoll et al. 1980) found that those being maintained on heroin did only moderately better than those receiving oral methadone. Another researcher notes, "While heroin-prescribed patients attended the clinic more regularly and showed some reduction in the extent of their criminal activities, nevertheless they showed no change in their other social activities such as work, stable accommodation or diet, nor did they differ significantly in the physical complications of drug use from those denied such a prescription" (Mitcheson 1994, 182). There was moderate leakage of heroin from the trial; 37 percent of those receiving heroin admitted that they at least occasionally sold some of their supply on the black market. An important factor in explaining the relatively weak results for heroin maintenance may have been the effort to limit doses. The average dose received by the patients, who had to bargain aggressively with their doctors, was 60 mg of pure heroin daily.[7]

Mostly, though, there has been indifference in Britain since the mid-1970s. This may in part reflect the much greater cost of providing heroin rather than methadone to a maintained patient. National Health Service reimbursement rules also make this more difficult for the practitioner. The claims of one British practitioner (John Marks, operating in the Liverpool metropolitan area) as to the efficacy of heroin in reducing criminal involvement aroused controversy and hostility, but little curiosity, in the British establishment. Observers from other nations, including Switzerland, were more interested (Ulrich-Votglin 1997).

THE SWISS HEROIN MAINTENANCE TRIALS

The Zurich government had attempted to deal with the city's severe heroin problem in the mid-1980s by allowing the operation of an open-air drug market behind the main train station. The Platzpitz was intended to minimize the intrusiveness of drug markets and to allow the efficient delivery of services, such as syringe exchange, to those who needed it. The city closed the Platzspitz in 1992 as a consequence of the in-migration of large numbers of heroin users from other parts of Switzerland and of the market's unsightliness (MacCoun and Reuter 2001, ch. 12).

Zurich authorities still sought an innovative approach, and in January 1994 they opened the first heroin maintenance clinics, part of a three-year national trial of heroin maintenance as a supplement to the large methadone maintenance program that had been operating for at least a decade. In late 1997 the federal government approved a large- scale expansion, which potentially would accommodate 15 percent of the nation's estimated thirty thousand heroin addicts.

The motivation for these trials was complex. Two federal officials suggested to us that it was partly an effort to forestall a strong legalization movement (personal communication, 1995). In their view, the Swiss citizenry were unwilling to be very tough about enforcement but also were offended by the unsightliness of the drug scene. Heroin maintenance was likely to reduce the visibility of the problem, arguably an important consideration in Swiss drug policy. A 1991 survey found that only about 10 percent favored police action against all drug users, but that 57 percent favored suppression of open drug scenes (Gutzwiller and Uchtenhagen 1997). For other policymaking participants, it was an obvious next step in reducing the risk of AIDS, which was very prevalent among intravenous drug users in Switzerland.

The decision was taken after very public consultations at the highest levels. An unusual "summit meeting" was held, at which the Swiss President and the heads of the cantonal governments approved an experiment to test whether heroin maintenance would reduce heroin problems.[8] Public opinion was generally supportive: in a 1991 poll, 72 percent expressed approval of controlled prescription of heroin (Gutzwiller and Uchtenhagen 1997).[9] The experiment was widely discussed in the media before implementation. An elaborate governance structure was established, including very detailed scrutiny by regional ethics officers (Uchtenhagen 1999). As an example of the care that was taken to protect the public health, enrollees were required to surrender their drivers' licenses, thus reducing the risk of their driving while heroin-intoxicated. Similarly, it was decided that once the government had provided heroin addicts with the drug, it incurred a continuing obligation to maintain those addicts as long as they sought heroin.

The original design involved three groups of patients receiving different injectable opiates: 250 got heroin, 250 got morphine, and 200 got methadone. The early experience with morphine was that it caused discomfort to the patients, and it was abandoned. Patients were reluctant to accept injectable methadone. As a consequence, the final report focused on injectable heroin.

Participants in the trials were required to be at least twenty years old, to have undergone two years of intravenous injecting, and to have failed at two other treatment attempts. These are hardly very tight screens. In fact, most of those admitted had extensive careers both in heroin addiction and in treatment. For example, in the Geneva site, the average age of participants was thirty-three, with twelve years of injecting heroin and eight prior treatment episodes.[10]

A decision to allow addicts to choose the dose they needed was critical. It removed any incentive to supplement the clinic provision with black-market purchases and eliminated a potentially important source of tension in the relationship with clinic personnel. A patient could receive heroin three times daily, 365 days of the year. The average daily dose was 500–600 mg of pure heroin, a massive amount by the standards of U.S. street addicts.[11] Faced with no constraint with respect to the drug that had dominated their lives and that had always been very difficult and expensive to obtain, patients initially sought very high doses. However, they quickly accepted more reasonable levels that still permitted many of them to function in everyday life, notwithstanding the relatively short-acting character of heroin.[12]

The patient self-injected with equipment prepared by the staff, who could also provide advice about injecting practices as they supervised the injection. There was a daily charge of 15 francs (ca. $10) to participants, many of whom paid out of their state welfare income. No heroin could be taken off the premises, thus minimizing the risk of leakage into the black market. Initially enrollment in the trials lagged behind schedule, but after the first year, enthusiasm among local officials increased sharply; consequently the trials ended up enlisting more than the initial targets and in a greater variety of settings than expected. Small towns (for example, St. Gallen) and prisons volunteered to be sites and were able to enroll clients. Nonetheless some sites, such as Geneva, were never able to reach their enrollment targets (Perneger et al. 1998).

The project certainly demonstrated the feasibility of heroin maintenance. By the end of the trials, over eight hundred patients had received heroin on a regular basis without leakage into the illicit market. No overdoses were reported among participants while they stayed in the program. The dosage levels ultimately chosen by the patients allowed many to improve their social and economic functioning.[13] A large majority of participants had maintained the regime that was imposed on them, requiring daily attendance at the clinic. For example, in Geneva twenty out of twenty-five patients received heroin on more than 80 percent of treatment days (Perneger et al. 1998).

Putting aside the question of appropriate controls, which we will address below, we can say that outcomes generally were very positive. Retention in treatment, a standard measure of treatment success, was high relative to rates found in methadone programs generally; 69 percent still were in treatment eighteen months after admission.[14] About half of those recorded as drop-outs in fact moved to other treatment modalities, some choosing methadone and others abstinence-based modalities. One observer suggested that having discovered the limitations of untrammeled access to heroin, these patients were now ready to attempt quitting.

Crime rates were much reduced, compared to those reported at treatment entry. Self-reported rates fell by 60 percent during the first six months, and this figure was supported by data from official arrest records. Self-reported use of nonprescribed heroin fell sharply. The percentage of participants with jobs that were described as "permanent" increased from 14 percent to 32 percent, while unemployment fell from 44 percent to 20 percent. Self-reported mental health also improved substantially.

Cocaine use remained high during heroin maintenance. Only three new HIV infections, probably related to cocaine use outside of the clinics, were detected. One interesting, albeit negative, finding is that though many addicts were able to detach themselves from the heroin subculture, they were unable to develop other attachments. In retrospect, given their weak labor force performance and their estrangement over a previous decade from nonaddicts, this should not be surprising. But it does point to the long-term challenge for psychosocial services.

The evaluation carried out by the Swiss government was led by Ambros Uchtenhagen, a leading Swiss drug treatment researcher. The trial design, which focused on comparing before-and-after behavior of the patients and which lacked a well-specified control group (Killias and Uchtenhagen 1996), limited the power of the findings. In the absence of a control group or of random assignment, the natural metric for assessing the program would have been the success of methadone programs with similar patients, yet the heroin maintenance trial participants were targeted with substantially more psychosocial services than was the typical methadone patient. Critics asked whether the claimed success was a function of using heroin or, rather, of the additional services (Farrell and Hall 1998). Another problem was that the evaluation relied primarily on self-reports by patients, with few objective measures included.

Only at the Geneva site was there random assignment between heroin maintenance and other modalities. Compared to the controls, during the trial period, experimental subjects in Geneva were substantially less involved in the street heroin markets, were less criminally active generally, and showed greater improvement in social functioning and mental health. On a number of other dimensions the two groups did not differ: both improved in measures of drug overdoses, precautions against AIDS, and overall health status. Unfortunately, the significance of the meticulous evaluation of that site was limited by a small sample size (twenty-five in the experimental group and twenty-two controls)—which biases analyses against rejecting the null hypothesis of "no difference"—and by a lack of reported detail on the treatments received by the controls.

In addressing the subject of controls, it is difficult to know what an appropriate control group would be for assessing these results in even a crude sense. The Swiss trials involved demonstration programs, which are likely to be undertaken by higher-quality program operators with more staff esprit, and to be administered with greater fidelity than are routine methadone maintenance programs. Possibly it is most appropriate to compare their outcomes with those of methadone maintenance when it was a new pharmacotherapy, in the early 1970s. Hall et al. (1998) note, in the same spirit, that programs which participate in randomized control trials of methadone maintenance show substantially higher retention rates than other programs.

Unsurprisingly, heroin maintenance turned out to be far more expensive than methadone maintenance. It required three-times-daily attendance and the provision of injecting equipment, while methadone is typically dispensed three times a week, with take-home doses for later consumption being allowed to most long-term patients. Moreover, the Swiss researchers report that it has, so far, been quite expensive to provide sufficient quantities of pure heroin, given that there previously was only a tiny legitimate market for the injectable form. The evaluators estimated total daily cost per patient at about 50 Swiss francs ($35), roughly twice the daily cost for a standard methadone program. Though the initial estimate of financial benefit per day of enrollment was 96 Swiss francs (including only savings on criminal investigations, jail stays, and health care costs), this hardly settles the matter of whether these additional costs are justified, particularly since most of the benefits accrue not to the health department but to a different government sector and to citizens directly.

More recently, Rehm et al. (2001) have reported results for the almost two thousand patients who entered heroin maintenance programs from the start of the trials in 1994 to the end of 2000, when the programs had been offered as a routine option for over two years. Not only does the treatment show very high retention rates by the standards of opiate programs, 70 percent for at least twelve months, but the dropout is primarily to other treatment modalities. Thirty-seven percent chose to transfer to a methadone maintenance program; another 22 percent chose an abstinence-based program. It seems increasingly plausible that such programs may persuade experienced users that untrammeled access to heroin does not eliminate all their life problems. Heroin maintenance may turn out, unexpectedly, to be a transitional modality.

RESPONSES TO THE SWISS TRIALS

Since political considerations are so central to this issue, the political response engendered by the Swiss trials both at home and abroad is interesting.

Domestically, the trials became the focus of the two extreme wings of Swiss opinion, which used the very open referendum process to propound their views.[15] One group, Youth Without Drugs, obtained enough signatures to place on the ballot a measure that would "exclude further controlled prescription experiments and methadone, end attempts to differentiate between soft and hard drugs and focus prevention programmes on deterrence only" (Klingemann 1996, 733). Shortly after the launching of the Youth Without Drugs initiative, an opposing group was created with the cumbersome name For a Reasonable Drug Policy—Tabula Rasa with the Drug Mafia. They advocated adding a new article to the Constitution stating that "the consumption, production, possession and purchase of narcotics for individual use only is not prohibited." They also obtained the one hundred thousand signatures necessary for putting their proposal on the ballot.

The federal government opposed both initiatives. In the vote on the abstinence initiative in September 1997, almost four years after the Youth Without Drugs group had gathered their signatures, 70 percent of voters rejected the proposition.[16] This strong majority provided important support for the government in its decision to extend the trials into a second phase. A referendum on the legalization initiative was handily defeated in November 1998.

The heroin trials also proved controversial internationally. The International Narcotics Control Board (INCB), a U.N. agency that, inter alia, regulates the international trade in legal opiates, very reluctantly authorized the importation of the heroin required for the trials (Klingemann 1996). The INCB required, when approving the initial importation of heroin, that the Swiss government agree to an independent evaluation by the World Health Organization, but that evaluation had still not appeared as of December 1998, even though the trials themselves were completed in December 1996 (McGregor 1998). When it did appear, the evaluation was critical of the research design but concluded that the trials showed the feasibility of heroin maintenance and resulting improvements in health and social functioning (Ali et al. 1999). The concluding sentence of the summary, however, points to the limited enthusiasm of the panel for the experiment: "There is need for continued skepticism about the specific benefits of one short acting opioid over others and there is a need for further studies to establish objectively the differences in the effect of these different opioids."

The INCB expressed concern about the proposed expansion of the trials (INCB 1998). The language used was unusually strong for a U.N. agency, especially one dealing not with a pariah country such as Afghanistan or Burma but with a veritable bulwark of international respectability and the home of the World Health Organization (WHO), among many other U.N. agencies. The director general of the INCB cautioned, "Anyone who plays with fire loses control over it." He also claimed that expanded heroin trials would send "a disastrous signal to countries in which drugs were produced"; those nations would ask why they should cut back cultivation "when the same drugs were being given out legally in Europe." The board's annual report more diplomatically regretted the proposed expansion of the scheme before the completion of the WHO evaluation.

The Swiss trials sparked interest in other wealthy nations. The Dutch government committed itself to launch a trial of injectable heroin for purposes of addiction maintenance (Maginnis 1997). This came after almost fifteen years of inconclusive discussions about such trials, following a rather murky episode in which the Amsterdam municipal health authority had attempted to maintain about forty addicts on morphine (Derks 1997). That Switzerland was willing to take on the disapproval of the international community was undoubtedly helpful in pushing the Dutch government to launch a trial involving 750 addicts. In Australia, the trials also helped spark interest in a feasibility study in Canberra, which has a substantial heroin addiction problem (Bammer and McDonald 1994). Only the personal intervention of the prime minister in 1997, overriding a decision by a council of state and federal ministers, prevented the study from moving to the next pilot stage. There have been expressions of interest from Denmark as well.

HEROIN MAINTENANCE IN THE UNITED STATES, POST-1950

Surprisingly, there was some discussion of a heroin maintenance trial in the United States during the period 1950–70, when heroin dependence was a fairly invisible, and probably minor, problem. Indeed, in 1957 the interim report of the joint Committee on Narcotic Study of the American Medical Association and the American Bar Association recommended exploring the possibility of an experiment in outpatient heroin maintenance (Bayer 1976). However, the most significant episode of modern times occurred in the early 1970s, near the height of the U.S. heroin epidemic, when serious consideration was given to a trial of heroin maintenance in New York City. Though the incident occurred so long ago, it is worth briefly describing because it illustrates the continuity, perhaps even stagnation, of drug policy debates (Judson 1974, 126–40).

The Vera Institute, then a young but already well respected social policy research institution with its roots primarily in criminal justice, initiated plans to test heroin maintenance in the United States, having been impressed by the apparent success of the British in keeping their heroin addict population to manageable numbers.[17] It proposed a pilot program for New York City in which addicts would be provided with heroin for an initial period of perhaps three months and then would be switched to methadone or to an abstinence regime. The rationale was to use the heroin as a means of persuading recalcitrant addicts to enter programs. If a first batch of thirty patients performed well in this regime, then a second set of two hundred would be selected and randomly assigned to either the same regime or methadone maintenance. Only then would a large-scale implementation be tried.

Though far from a long-term heroin maintenance scheme, this proposal generated extremely hostile reactions from all quarters. Harlem's congressman Charles Rangel said, "It is imperative that we dispel some of the myths about the British system of drug treatment so that the American people will open up their eyes and recognize heroin for what it is—a killer, not a drug on which a human being should be maintained." The head of the predecessor agency to DEA asserted, "It would be a virtual announcement of medical surrender on the treatment of addiction and would amount to consigning hundreds of thousands of our citizens to the slavery of heroin addiction forever." Vincent Dole, one of the two developers of methadone, published an editorial in the *Journal of the American Medical Association* attacking the notion on many grounds, including the impossibility of finding stable doses and the implausibility that such a small-scale demonstration could establish the feasibility of providing services to 250,000 heroin users. Even the reliably liberal *New York Times* published negative coverage, for example, citing a Swedish psychiatric epidemiologist who argued: "You could easily get up to three or four million addicts in five years. Heroin maintenance? Only those who don't know anything about addiction can discuss it" (quotes from Judson 1974, 131–32).

Each of these quoted critics could be discounted for representing a specific interest group or bias. Rangel represented the hardest-hit population group, African-Americans, who had a deep suspicion that drugs were being employed to reduce black anger following the urban riots of the late 1960s. Law enforcement agencies are notoriously conservative. The researcher responsible for developing a substitute medication for heroin was hardly likely to be an enthusiast for returning to the original drug. And Sweden was, as a nation, harshly anti-maintenance, even against methadone. But, with so many different enemies, ultimately the proposal had no friends. It simply disappeared.

A few years later the National League of Cities considered endorsing trials of heroin maintenance in several cities. After much debate, it reaffirmed its support for such trials but, as Senay et al. report, "thereafter the topic receded into obscurity" (1996, 192). Later research proposals also died. David Lewis, a participant in the original Vera proposal, attributes the defeats to perceived problems with their scientific merit (Senay et al. 1996), a view that Charles O'Brien, a member of the peer review committee, confirms (personal communication). In one case, however, the NIDA National Council, intended to advise NIDA on policy issues, overruled the approval of a scientific panel (Senay et al. 1996).

In the United States political reaction to the Swiss trials was illustrated by hearings held by a House subcommittee. The subcommittee called as witnesses two doctors from Switzerland with long records of hostility to both needle exchange and heroin maintenance. One, Ernst Aeschbach, was on the board of Youth Without Drugs. The other, Erne Mathias, asserted that there was a conspiracy, initially supported by the East German or Soviet intelligence agency, to create "narco states." In Europe, he claimed, Switzerland had been targeted when the Netherlands acquired too controversial a reputation. Most members, both Democratic and Republican, were delighted with the Swiss physicians, who were supported by two hawkish U.S. witnesses who also condemned the trials. In introducing the hearing, Representative Dennis Hastert (R-Ill.) had commented, "Giving away free needles or doctor-injected heroin is simply . . . a fast track to moral corruption and the first step towards genuine disintegration of public security." No Swiss researcher or official associated with the trials was given an opportunity to testify.

Still the proposal recurs. David Vlahov, a professor at the Johns Hopkins School of Public Health, proposed once again in 1998 to undertake a trial. The usual chorus of disapproval was instantaneous. Maryland's Democratic governor said, "It doesn't make any sense. It sends totally the wrong signal." The lieutenant governor expanded on this slightly: "It's much better to tell young people that heroin is bad. This undermines the whole effort." Even Mayor of Baltimore Kurt Schmoke, a leader in liberal drug policy, distanced himself from the proposal and censured his health commissioner for endorsing it. A leading newspaper reported that "many addiction experts say funding for traditional drug treatment falls far short of the demand, and heroin maintenance is a dubious distraction from proven remedies for drug abuse" (quotes from *Baltimore Sun*, June 12, 1998).

SHOULD THE UNITED STATES INITIATE A HEROIN MAINTENANCE TRIAL?

Perhaps the principal accomplishment of the Swiss trials was simply to show that heroin maintenance is possible, a matter that previously had been in question. For example, Kaplan (1983) doubted the feasibility of even an experiment in heroin maintenance and raised a host of possible objections, from community rejection of sites at which addicts might be found nodding off (p. 175) to heroin diversion by employees. The Swiss have shown that— at least in the context of a wealthy, well-ordered society—it is possible to maintain, in a way that the community finds acceptable, large numbers of addicts with previously chaotic lives, and to do so without any dire consequences to the health and safety of the community or of participants. Indeed, the addicts' ability to operate in society appears to have been enhanced.

Normative Issues

Feasibility, however, does not imply desirability. Heroin maintenance has a contradiction at its heart. Having chosen to prohibit the drug, society then makes an exception for those who cause sufficient damage to themselves and society as a consequence of their violation of the prohibition. Society must decide on the damage level that entitles a user to access. Addicts may be required to cause a lot of damage in order to gain access. That approach is expensive (in terms of crime and health risks) and seems inhumane. Alternatively, if the damage barrier is set low, then access to heroin becomes too easy, and the basic prohibition may be substantially weakened.

Linked to this quandary is a revulsion against the government providing the prohibited drug. A purely private market would probably raise far fewer objections but is implausible. The impoverished condition of so many American heroin addicts and society's desire to require that the drug be provided in the context of other services, such as employment training and counseling, mean that the state will certainly have a central role in the funding and regulation of heroin maintenance, if not in its provision. Thus heroin maintenance is more troubling than merely removing a restriction on the right of private provision of the drug.

We present this as a normative argument, distinct both from the political issue of whether such a role can obtain popular support and the related argument that heroin maintenance would reduce the effectiveness of the basic prohibition by "sending the wrong signal" (MacCoun 1998). The state has moral as well as programmatic purposes; providing a prohibited substance that has caused so much harm will appear to some as normatively inconsistent, no matter what benefits it yields. Similar normative concerns are often voiced about the inconsistency of current policies toward alcohol, tobacco, and other drugs, though to little effect.

In highlighting this problem, we should also identify a potential misunderstanding. The question of whether "normatively inconsistent" messages would lead to increased drug use and drug-related harms is one that can be answered empirically, and the Swiss trials and any possible U.S. trials would be relevant sources of data. On the other hand, the view discussed above— that inconsistent government messages are intrinsically undesirable (irrespective of their consequences)—is a purely normative matter that no empirical study can address.

Heroin maintenance presents other conceptual problems. Providing heroin in accord with the desires of the patient may allow for the delivery of psychosocial services that do indeed assist the addict in dealing with his or her problem. But a case can be made that heroin maintenance is of itself social policy, not medicine. Indeed, the INCB's objections to authorizing the shipments of opiates to Switzerland emphasized just that point. Arguably, interventions that blur the boundaries between social policy and therapeutic treatment exploit and perhaps weaken the bonds of legitimacy and trust that underpin the medical relationship.

These are issues that can be addressed without an American field trial. For some decision makers they are troubling considerations that might nonetheless be waived if it were shown that the reductions in disease and crime were large enough. But other decision makers might feel that there are no findings of efficacy that could surmount the obstacles presented by these moral concerns—though it should be noted that similar objections against methadone largely gave way in the face of overwhelming evidence of reduced criminality, morbidity, and mortality.

Political Considerations

Another class of concerns that vitiate the need for a trial is political. Methadone advocates and researchers express a concern that heroin maintenance would undermine public support for maintenance therapy more generally, in particular for methadone. New York Mayor Giuliani's August 1998 attack on methadone maintenance for its failure to move addicts to abstinence is a reminder of how thin is the foundation of public understanding on which those programs rest, notwithstanding that he backed away from this position six months later. After all, only ten years before, the White House Conference on Drug Abuse (1988) had produced a report that opposed methadone maintenance. A population that doubts the morality of providing such a relatively unattractive narcotic as methadone is likely to be extremely skeptical about providing the demonized heroin. If heroin were to be offered, then methadone maintenance might come under renewed attack.

Wayne Hall argues that in Australia the controversy over a small-scale heroin maintenance trial in Canberra has given new ammunition to those who oppose both methadone maintenance and needle exchange (Hall, personal communication, 1998). It is easy to caricature the idea of heroin maintenance, and that caricature rubs off on programs that have the similar goal of reducing drug-related problems without a focus on simply persuading or forcing addicts to quit using habit-forming illegal drugs. Moreover, the claim of a heroin "crisis" that served earlier as justification for taking a trial seriously may have backfired by inadvertently giving support to calls for greater toughness against addicts in a country that often waves the banner of harm reduction over its drug policies.

A related political argument focuses on the allocation of research resources. The budget for treatment innovations is limited; one can reasonably question whether, given the political obstacles to heroin maintenance, the marginal dollar should go into trials of a program that is unlikely to be implemented. This is certainly a conservative view of social innovation generally. A research program on heroin maintenance is clearly a long-term effort. Predicting the political climate for maintenance ten years in the future is a very risky enterprise.

The Swiss experience demonstrates that in a wealthy society which values order and sobriety, it is possible to build a base of popular support for heroin maintenance. On the other hand, Switzerland is a somewhat paternalistic society, and its citizens may be less troubled than are individualistic-minded Americans by some of the normative issues discussed here, though there is little positive evidence to support that speculation. Segalman (1986) describes the Swiss welfare system as mixed in this respect. The United States has much more of an ideology of individualism and distaste for state support generally. But one can pose the political question in a more positive light: What can one learn from Switzerland about how to build popular support for a heroin maintenance trial?

Programmatic Concerns

National stereotypes are an important consideration in the argument for a U.S. trial. Americans see Switzerland as a fairly homogeneous and orderly society, where program operators can be trusted and even heroin addicts are probably given to following rules. Though Swiss addicts in fact have high rates of criminality, they are (like European addicts and criminals generally) vastly less violent than their American counterparts. Also, the kind of fraud that has characterized the U.S. methadone industry from time to time is at least not reported in Switzerland and is not raised as a serious problem even by methadone opponents. Thus there would be the need for a demonstration to determine whether, inter alia, American program operators could be monitored and coerced effectively enough to guarantee that diversion would be a minor problem, and whether American addicts would be capable of meeting the demands imposed by a three-times-a-day clinic attendance requirement.

Such a trial could be structured to answer a charge of some critics that heroin maintenance is simply not an important policy innovation because it will bring in few addicts not currently in treatment (Farrell and Hall 1998). The initial Swiss recruitment difficulties suggest that few addicts will enter heroin maintenance programs voluntarily, no matter how attractive they sound in theory. For example, the Geneva site found that only one member of the control group moved to the heroin program when access was provided. Conducting the trials in smaller cities, where they could reach a significant proportion of the total heroin addict population, would permit a clearer assessment of their attractiveness.

Ironically, one piece of evidence that puritan critics are incorrect in claiming that these programs amount to providing whiskey to alcoholics is that they have not proved attractive enough to the intended clients to make much of a difference. Drug programs theoretically can be effective and immoral or ineffective and moral. The maintenance regime, with its highly routinized provision of the mythologized drug in a sterile environment, may fall in between for most heroin addicts. It takes the glamour from the drug that has dominated their lives, without providing any cure for their addiction. Informal inquiries among Zurich addicts early in the trial elicited the response that heroin maintenance was a program for "losers" (Hall, personal communication). It may do little more than improve the performance of a small fraction of those who would otherwise choose methadone but prove erratic participants in that modality. The second-stage, expanded Swiss program will help to answer that question.

Even if the evaluation results hold up on tighter inspection and heroin outperforms methadone in terms of improving health and reducing crime among participants, some important empirical questions about population effects may remain unanswered. The Swiss evaluation has been patient-focused. This focus elides one of the basic concerns of opponents: that broad availability of heroin maintenance will increase the attractiveness of heroin use, or even of drug use more generally. Answering that question requires more than pilot programs, since it is precisely a function of scale. Evaluations of small-scale pilot projects have inherent limits, a point made by Vincent Dole (1972) in the context of the Vera initiative. Again, that observation argues for trials in a smaller city, where experimental programs might have observable effects on the general population.

It is worth noting that large-scale expansion of heroin maintenance, if it substantially reduces addict involvement in heroin use and selling, may actually have the benign effect of making heroin less accessible to new users. Markets are now primarily supplied at the retail level by long-term addicts; if these mostly withdraw, then nonaddicted users, particularly experimenters, may have difficulty finding a regular source.[18] One can argue that the reduction in harmfulness might make heroin use more attractive (see MacCoun 1998). In particular, someone who initiates with black-market heroin when heroin maintenance is available might reason that if he or she does become dependent, the habit will be supported by doses of predictable purity and potency, at a modest price and from a reliable and safe source.

At the margin, this is possible. It is hard, though, to imagine someone with the foresightedness to reason this way who would knowingly choose to become "enslaved" to a drug, no matter the available source. Moreover, such a person would have to knowingly accept the substantial risks of using black-market heroin for a period of years before becoming eligible for a maintenance program. One might also argue that heroin maintenance would reduce the likelihood that an addict would become abstinent. We find this compelling in the abstract, but the argument loses some of its force when one considers the remarkably long duration of heroin "careers" in the current system (see, e.g., Hser et al. 1993) . At any rate, such prevalence-increasing effects might be counterbalanced by the substantial reduction in black-market access that would result when current addicts stop frequenting, and running, those markets.

CONCLUSION

The harshness of reactions in the international community to the Swiss trials illustrates the difficulty faced by nations interested in testing harm-reduction innovations. The other much-disapproved-of harm reduction innovation is the Dutch coffee shops, which can legally sell small amounts of marijuana and hashish to anyone over age eighteen. These shops could arguably be viewed as undercutting the sovereignty of neighboring countries because they provide easy access for French and German citizens otherwise prohibited from buying these drugs (Korf and Riper 1999). In contrast, the Swiss heroin maintenance programs were clearly restricted to that nation's own citizens. Rather than responding with enthusiasm to the promising findings of the trials, many observers seized upon the undoubted weaknesses of the evaluation to accuse trial supporters of social irresponsibility. There was no recognition that current policies—in particular, the tough enforcement of prohibitions—have a much thinner research base beneath them. Aggressive crackdowns, even if they result in no demonstrable benefits and do cause highly visible harms in terms of increased violence, are immune from such international condemnation.

What is so striking here is that all this hostility is engendered not by a policy idea but simply by a proposal to conduct a demonstration or trial. Clearly there are serious ethical issues involved in government provision of a prohibited drug. Though it is not precisely a slippery slope, heroin maintenance goes farther down a path started by methadone maintenance and needle exchange, two programs we endorse heartily. We confess to some squeamishness about heroin maintenance. It is easier to feel than to articulate the qualitative breakpoint between it and the other two programs. Needle exchange and methadone maintenance each help addicts meet their need in a safer way. Methadone maintenance does so in a way that is less pleasurable than injecting heroin, but that is not true of needle exchange. Still, providing a full rather than an empty needle seems a substantial step, perhaps because needles of themselves are so often seen as benign, the source of cure rather than illness. One can object to facilitating pleasure on either consequentialist or deontological grounds.

Even some of the empirical objections to heroin maintenance cannot readily be answered through a small-scale trial in a very large city. But it is still difficult to account for the indignation and the willful misrepresentation of foreign experiences (Britain in the 1970s; Switzerland in the 1990s). If a substantial percentage of current heroin addicts were to participate, which is by no means certain, heroin maintenance might well result in large gains in health, social functioning, and criminal justice costs.

We return to our initial point. Society's tools for alleviating the problems of heroin addiction are weak. Heroin maintenance offers some prospect of helping. It is worth serious consideration, certainly more than the hasty dismissal that it routinely receives from so many participants, researchers included.

ACKNOWLEDGMENTS

This essay is taken from Robert MacCoun and Peter Reuter, *Drug War Heresies: Learning from Other Vices, Times, and Places* (New York: Cambridge University Press, 2001), where it appears in slightly different form. Financial support for the research reported here was provided by the Alfred P. Sloan Foundation through a grant to the Drug Policy Research Center at RAND. We have benefited from discussion with Michael Farrell and Wayne Hall.

NOTES

1. As an indication of methadone's global reach, at least among wealthy nations of predominantly European-origin population, the best book-length review of methadone treatment is from Australia: Ward et al. (1998).

2. For example, Hall et al. (1998, 46) cite studies showing no more than 50 percent in treatment even six months after entry. The classic study of methadone programs, showing the wide range of services delivered and outcomes achieved, is Ball and Ross (1991).

3. Hser et al. (1993) report on a twenty-four-year follow-up of a cohort of heroin addicts recruited in 1962–64. They found that of those interviewed in 1986, only 20 percent reported having been abstinent from heroin during the past three years.

4. Musto (1999, ch.7) provides a good account of the operation of these clinics and of the federal efforts to close them.

5. The British long have complained about foreign descriptions of their system and, in particular, of the nature of the 1967 changes (Strang and Gossop 1994). The nuances of a system largely dependent on informal social controls are difficult to capture. Pearson (1991) provides a succinct version. Stimson and Oppenheimer (1982, ch. 6) give a fuller account. For current practice, see Strang et al. 1996.

6. Trebach (1982, ch. 7) provides an interesting account of why the shift to

oral methadone occurred, emphasizing the discomfort of medical personnel with supporting the act of injection.

7. On the struggles between patient and doctor, see Edwards 1969.

8. The Swiss presidency is not an extremely august position: it is occupied in six-month rotations by each member of the seven-person cabinet elected by the Parliament. Nevertheless, the President does represent the leadership of the federal government.

9. Interestingly, a later administration of the same survey found a noticeable increase in the percentage opposing controlled prescription between 1991 and 1994 (from 24 to 30 percent): this was a period during which the trials were being debated publicly.

10. The final results of the evaluation were published in Uchtenhagen 1999. We use more detailed data from individual sites.

11. At $1 per milligram, a low street price in recent years outside of New York, that would amount to $500–$600 per day in heroin expenditures alone. The actual daily expenditure figure in the mid-1990s was about one-tenth of that.

12. A telling comment on these dynamics is provided by Haemmig (1995, 377): "People in the project tend to take too much of the drug. Many seem to have a concept that their only real problem in life is to get enough drugs. In the projects, for the first time in their lives, they can have as much as they need. In the course of time it gets depressing for them to realize that they have problems other than just getting enough drugs."

13. The Geneva site reported that they reached stable doses within the first month.

14. Eighteen months was chosen as the assessment period because only a modest fraction had entered treatment more than eighteen months before the agreed-upon termination date for the trials as such.

15. "The Swiss vote in more referendums than anyone else. Each year they are asked three or four times to take part in national votes—not to mention referendums in the cantons and communes" (*Economist*, October 17, 1998, 58).

16. An earlier referendum, confined to Zurich and focused merely on the continuation of funding for the pilot scheme, was approved by over 60 percent of the voters ("Swiss Voters Approve Heroin Distribution Program," Associated Press, December 1, 1996).

17. Judson (1974) reports that a Vera research group originally had viewed the British maintenance regimes negatively and had projected very large increases in the number of addicts. When those increases were not realized, they changed their view of the British programs.

18. Treatment also has this effect, drawing from markets individuals who are both users and sellers, thus simultaneously affecting demand and supply. For an analysis of this phenomenon, see Caulkins et al. 1997.

REFERENCES

Ali, Robert, Marc Auriacombe, Miguel Casas, Linda Cottler, Michael Farrell, Dieter Kleiber, Arthur Kreuzer, Alan Ogborne, Jurgen Rehm, and Patricia Ward.

1999. Report of the External Panel on the Evaluation of the Swiss Scientific Studies of Medically Prescribed Narcotics to Drug Addicts. World Health Organization [WHO].

Ball, J., and A. Ross. 1991. *The Effectiveness of Methadone Maintenance Treatment: Patients, Programs, Services and Outcomes*. New York: Springer-Verlag.

Bammer, G., and D. McDonald. 1994. "Report on a Workshop on Trial Evaluation." In *Issues for Designing and Evaluating a "Heroin Trial."* Working Paper no. 8, Canberra, Australia: National Center for Epidemiology and Population Health.

Bayer, R. 1976. "Heroin Maintenance: An Historical Perspective on the Exhaustion of Liberal Narcotics Reform." *Journal of Psychedelic Drugs* 8: 157–65.

Caulkins, J., C. P. Rydell, W. Schwab, and J. Chiesa. 1997. *Mandatory Minimum Sentences: Throwing Away the Key or the Taxpayer's Money*. Santa Monica, Calif.: RAND.

Derks, J. 1997. "The Dispensing of Injectable Morphine in Amsterdam: Experiences, Results and Implications for the Swiss Project for the Medical Prescription of Narcotics." In Lewis et al. 1997, pp. 167–79.

Dole, Vincent. 1972. Editorial. *JAMA* 220: 1493.

Edwards, G. 1969. "The British Approach to the Treatment of Heroin Addiction." *Lancet* 1: 768–72.

Farrell, M., and W. Hall. 1998. "The Swiss Heroin Trials: Testing Alternative Approaches." *British Medical Journal* 316 (February 28): 639.

Gutzwiller, F., and A. Uchtenhagen. 1997. "Heroin Substitution: Part of the Fight Against Drug Dependency." In Lewis et al. 1997.

Haemmig, R. B. 1995. "Harm Reduction in Bern: From Outreach to Heroin Maintenance." *Bulletin of the New York Academy of Medicine* (Winter): 371–79.

Hall, W., R. Mattick, R. Ward, and J. Ward. 1998. "The Effectiveness of Methadone Maintenance Treatment 1: Heroin Use and Crime." In Ward et al. 1998, pp. 17–58.

Hartnoll, R., et al. 1980. "Evaluation of Heroin Maintenance in a Controlled Trial." *Archives of General Psychiatry* 37: 877–84.

Hser, Y.-I., M. D. Anglin, and K. Powers. 1993. "A Twenty-four-Year Follow-up of California Narcotics Addicts." *Archives of General Psychiatry* 50: 577–84.

International Narcotics Control Board (INCB). 1998. *Report of the International Narcotics Control Board for 1997*. Vienna: INCB.

Johnson, B. 1975. "Understanding British Addiction Statistics." *Bulletin on Narcotics* 27, no. 1: 49–66.

———. 1977. "How Much Heroin Maintenance (Containment) in Britain?" *International Journal of Addictions* 12: 361–98.

Judson, H. 1974. *Heroin Addiction in Britain: What Americans Can Learn from the English Experience*. New York: Harcourt Brace Jovanovich.

Kaplan, J. 1983. *The Hardest Drug: Heroin and Public Policy*. Chicago: University of Chicago Press.

Killias, M., and A. Uchtenhagen. 1996. "Does Medical Prescription Reduce Delinquency Among Drug-Addicts? On the Evaluation of the Swiss Heroin Prescription Project and Its Methodology." *Studies on Crime and Crime Prevention* 5: 245–56.

Klingemann, K. K. 1996. "Drug Treatment in Switzerland: Harm Reduction, Decentralization and Community Response." *Addiction* 91: 723–36.

Korf, D., and H. Riper. 1999. "Windmills in Their Minds? Drug Policy and Drug Research in the Netherlands." *Journal of Drug Issues* 29, no. 3: 451–72.

Lewis, D., C. Gear, M. Laubli Loud, and D. Langenick-Cartwright, eds. 1997. *The Medical Prescription of Narcotics: Scientific Foundations and Practical Experiences.* Seattle: Hogrefe and Huber.

MacCoun, R. 1998. "The Psychology of Harm Reduction." *American Psychologist* 53: 1199–1208.

MacCoun, R., and P. Reuter. 2001. *Drug War Heresies: Learning from Other Places, Other Times, and Other Vices,* New York: Cambridge University Press.

McGregor, A. 1998. "WHO Accused of Slowness in Evaluating Swiss Heroin-Addiction Treatment." *Lancet* 351: 891.

Maginnis, R. L. 1997. *Night Gallery: Heroin Giveaways Go Global.* Family Research Council. http://www.frc.org/insight/is97j1dr.html.

Mitcheson, M. 1994. "Drug Clinics in the 1970s." In Strang and Gossop, 1994.

Musto, D. 1999. *The American Disease: Origins of Narcotic Control.* 3d ed. New York: Oxford University Press.

Pearson, G. 1991. "Drug Control Policies in Britain." In Tonry 1991.

Perneger, T. V., F. Giner, M. del Rio, and A. Mno. 1998. "Randomised Trial of Heroin Maintenance Programme for Addicts Who Fail in Conventional Drug Treatments." *British Medical Journal* 317: 13–18.

Rehm, J.; P. Gshwend; T. Steffen; F. Gutzwiller; A. Dobler-Mikola; and A. Uchtenhagen. 2001. "Feasibility, Safety, and Efficacy of Injectable Heroin Prescription for Refractory Opioid Addicts: A Follow Up Study." *Lancet* 358: 1417–1420.

Rettig, R., and A. Yarmolinsky, eds. 1995. *Federal Regulation of Methadone Programs.* Washington, D.C.: National Academy Press.

Segalman, R. 1986. "Welfare and Dependency in Switzerland." *Public Interest* 82: 106–21.

Spear, B. 1994. "The Early Years of the 'British System' in Practice." In Strang and Gossop, 1994.

Stears, A. 1997. "The British Drug Treatment System: Personal Perspectives." In Lewis et al. 1997, 122–29.

Strang, J., and M. Gossop. 1994. "The 'British System': Visionary Anticipation or Masterly Inactivity?" In Strang and Gossop, 1994.

Strang, J., and M. Gossop, eds. 1994. *Heroin Addiction and Drug Policy: The British System.* Oxford: Oxford University Press.

Stimson, G., and E. Oppenheimer. 1982. *Heroin Addiction: Treatment and Control in Britain.* New York: Tavistock.

Tonry, M. 1991. *Crime and Justice: A Review of Research.* Vol. 14. Chicago: University of Chicago Press.

Trebach, A. S. 1982. *The Heroin Solution.* New Haven, Conn.: Yale University Press.

Uchtenhagen, A., ed. 1999. *Prescription of Narcotics for Heroin Addicts: Main Results of the Swiss National Cohort Study.* Vol. 1 of *Medical Prescription of Narcotics.* Basel and New York: Karger.

Ulrich-Vogtlin, U. 1997. "An Overview of the Projects." In Lewis et al. 1997, 76–79.

Ward, J., R. Mattick, and W. Hall, eds. 1998. *Methadone Maintenance Treatment and Other Opioid Replacement Therapies.* Amsterdam: Academic Press.

White House Conference on a Drug Free America. 1988. *The White House Conference for a Drug Free America: Final Report, June 1988.* Washington, D.C.: U.S. Government Printing Office.

11

From Heroin Addiction to Opioid Maintenance: Problem or Cure? Or, All Opioid Agonists Are Not the Same

Richard S. Schottenfeld

There has been considerable discussion recently about proposals, coming from opposite ends of the political spectrum, to reduce public support for methadone maintenance or to institute heroin maintenance treatment for heroin dependence. These proposals point to ongoing controversy about the goals of addiction treatment and to misunderstanding or lack of clarity about the mechanisms of action and effectiveness of maintenance treatment. Curiously enough, these very different proposals are based on a similar rationale. Mayor Rudolph Giuliani in New York called for an end to methadone maintenance because maintaining heroin addicts on one substance that binds to brain opiate receptors and activates them (that is, an opioid agonist) is viewed as no better than keeping them addicted to another. Proponents of heroin maintenance—arguing from a similar premise that there is virtually no difference between heroin and methadone—call for implementation of heroin maintenance to increase the market penetration of maintenance treatment, which is viewed as the most effective response to heroin addiction.

My thesis, stated as the subtitle of this article, is that not all opioid agonists are the same, or equal, and that an understanding of the mechanisms of action and effectiveness of opiate-agonist maintenance treatment should, though probably won't, inform policy debates. I would like to review the rationales for opioid-agonist maintenance treatment, to discuss four medications used for maintenance treatment (methadone, naltrexone, levo-acetyl alpha methadol [LAAM], and buprenorphine), all of which target the mu opiate receptor, and to review the evidence regarding the effective ingredients of maintenance treatment. Then I will discuss some of the problems and limitations of current maintenance treatment in the United States and the policy and program options for addressing these issues.

AGONIST AND ANTAGONIST EFFECTS

The rationale for maintenance treatment presupposes that heroin addiction is perpetuated by a number of factors (Dole 1988). First, once addicted, subjects use heroin to relieve acute or protracted withdrawal symptoms (a negative reinforcement). Second, addicts use heroin because they have cravings for it or the compulsion to use it. Craving is a complex (and incompletely understood) neurobiologic, cognitive, and emotional state. It may be related to withdrawal, priming, or classical conditioning. "Priming" is a term that refers to the appetizing effects of sampling a substance: it's easier to avoid eating the first potato chip than it is to stop after trying one. Conditioned cues, such as visiting a "copping" place or seeing the drug, also may precipitate craving, possibly through the same brain pathways that mediate priming. The compulsion to use heroin may reflect long-lasting or even permanent changes in brain reward pathways and memory systems resulting from repeated heroin use or dependence.

Third, addicts use heroin to get high and to relieve psychological or emotional distress; positive and negative reinforcements perpetuate heroin addiction. And fourth, social factors encourage heroin use. These include peer influence, heroin availability, and stressful life situations, such as seemingly inescapable poverty or, at one time, military service in Vietnam.

The pharmacologic effects of methadone maintenance, or, more generally, of opioid agonist maintenance treatment—that is, sustaining an addict at a steady-state level of a medication that binds to and activates the mu receptor—address the first three of these four factors. First, continuous, steady-state opioid maintenance prevents withdrawal. Second, craving and the compulsion to use heroin are relieved during opioid agonist maintenance treatment at sufficiently high doses (Dole 1988). Reduction in craving may result from preventing withdrawal and also from maintaining a satiated state: it's easier to eat only one potato chip when you're not hungry. Finally, gradual increase in the dose of the opioid agonist during maintenance treatment leads to the development of tolerance to opioids, so that the euphoric effects of street heroin doses are blocked or attenuated.

Opioid agonist maintenance also may reduce psychological and emotional distress for some individuals. Thus, opioid agonist maintenance treatment eliminates or significantly reduces virtually all of the reinforcing pharmacologic effects of heroin use. From a learning theory perspective, this absence of reinforcement will lead to extinguishing the associated behavior, heroin self-administration. Other, nonpharmacologic, aspects of opioid agonist maintenance treatment programs, including the program structure and rules and the counseling components, target the social factors perpetuating use and thereby contribute substantially to the overall effectiveness of the treatment (McLellan et al. 1993; Ball and Ross 1991).

The pharmacologic targets of maintenance treatment with an opioid *antagonist* are limited to the second and third of the factors perpetuating addiction—reducing craving and blocking the continued positive reinforcement associated with heroin use (Rounsaville 1995). Naltrexone, for instance, binds tightly to the mu opioid receptor but has no intrinsic activity there. Since the affinity of naltrexone at the mu receptor is approximately 100 times greater than the affinity of heroin or morphine, in the presence of naltrexone, heroin is competitively inhibited from binding to and activating the receptor. Thus, during naltrexone maintenance, addicts experience little or no euphoria or other positive effects from heroin use, and this generally leads to curtailment of use of the drug, extinguishing the behavior.

Craving typically is reduced when drugs are not available, such as on a deserted island or in a controlled, drug-free setting. Consequently, antagonist maintenance treatment, which makes heroin unavailable to the brain, also reduces craving (Meyer and Mirin 1979). In addition, there is evidence suggesting that priming is mediated by opiate activity in the brain. If so, naltrexone may then block craving by blocking priming. In this model, with naltrexone it might be less tempting to try the first potato chip and also easier to stop after one. Recently, naltrexone has been found effective as a treatment for alcohol dependence. It may decrease some of the pleasurable effects of alcohol that are mediated in the brain by naturally occurring opioids (endorphins). Blocking opiate-mediated priming may be another mechanism underlying its effectiveness for alcohol as well as for opiate dependence (O'Malley et al. 1992). As with opioid agonist maintenance treatment, counseling components are needed in an antagonist maintenance program to address social, psychological, and emotional factors contributing to addiction and relapse.

Despite the theoretical promise of antagonist maintenance treatment, it has not been nearly as effective or widely used in clinical practice as opioid agonist treatment for a number of reasons. First, addicts need to be withdrawn from heroin prior to initiation of treatment—otherwise, drugs like naltrexone will precipitate such severe withdrawal symptoms that patients will never return for continued treatment. In addition, following withdrawal, heroin addicts may continue to experience mild symptoms of opiate withdrawal and mood disturbances, which may be related to changes in brain structure and function caused by heroin addiction. Relapse rates are high during the waiting period following heroin discontinuation and preceding initiation of nal-trexone treatment. Finally, because opioid antagonists are not inherently reinforcing, and patients can discontinue naltrexone use, for instance, with-out experiencing withdrawal symptoms, medication compliance and reten-tion in treatment tend to be quite low.

Development of sustained-release formulations (necessitating only monthly administration to maintain opiate blockade), or discovery of medi-cations that can reverse or ameliorate persistent withdrawal symptoms and mood disturbances associated with protracted abstinence, could lead to im-proved antagonist maintenance treatment outcomes. Given the complexity, variety, and specific locations of the changes in brain structure and function caused by heroin addiction, it is doubtful that we will soon find a single magic bullet that can reset all of the changes (Nestler 1992). Aversive contingen-cies, such as threatened revocation of a medical license for an addicted phy-sician and revocation of probation or parole for an addict under supervision of the criminal justice system, have been used successfully to increase com-pliance and retention (Rounsaville 1995; Cornish et al. 1997). Nevertheless, very few heroin addicts are maintained on naltrexone.

METHADONE VERSUS HEROIN MAINTENANCE

One might think that any opioid agonist would be as effective as any other for agonist maintenance treatment, and this belief, of course, serves as one of the principal rationales for proposing heroin maintenance. However, there are a number of differences between methadone and heroin, and a number of advantages in substituting methadone for heroin in maintenance treat-ment.

First, methadone is effective orally, so a less dangerous route of adminis-tration is substituted for the more dangerous practice of injection. Oral ad-ministration also leads to a more gradual rate of rise in plasma and brain opioid levels. Since the rate of rise is associated with the intensity of eupho-ria, or rush, associated with drug use, oral ingestion of methadone produces less powerful positive reinforcement than intravenous, smoked, or intranasal heroin use.

Second, methadone is long-acting: it needs to be administered only once a day, while heroin must be used at least two to three times each day to pre-vent withdrawal. Substituting a longer-acting for a shorter-acting opioid re-duces the amount of time an addict must focus on obtaining and using drugs. Even longer-acting opioids, such as LAAM and buprenorphine, which need to be administered only three times per week, may further reduce the addict's preoccupation with drug use, which is one of the hallmarks of addiction.

Third, on ingestion, methadone is widely distributed in tissues and organs throughout the body, including, most importantly, the liver. While methadone has no toxic effects on body functioning, even when used continuously for many decades, the liver serves as a reservoir for the drug, so that methadone plasma levels fluctuate within a relatively small range throughout the day. In contrast, heroin plasma levels fluctuate much more widely in relation to repeated use. With heroin use, addicts generally experience repeated cycles of incipient withdrawal, characterized by anxiety and early physical withdrawal symptoms, followed by symptom relief and a rush associated with heroin use, some period of a dreamlike state or "nod," return to normal mood, and then, once again, incipient withdrawal (Meyer and Mirin 1979). Even with uninterrupted access to the drug, in laboratory settings, chronic heroin self-administration led to increased psychopathology and dysphoria (Meyer and Mirin 1979). Reports from some of the current clinical trials of heroin maintenance document cognitive impairments associated with heroin administration (Petitjean et al. 2000).

With methadone maintenance, the daily oral dose leads to a gradual rise in plasma levels over a two-hour period and then a gradual reduction in plasma levels over the next twenty-two hours. These changes are generally associated with no or very little effect on mood or cognitive function either immediately following the daily dose or during the following twenty-four hours until the next dose. Of considerable importance, and possibly related to maintaining relatively steady-state plasma and brain methadone levels, methadone maintenance treatment leads to normalization of neuroendocrine and immune system functioning, which are disrupted by heroin addiction (Novick 1989). Gradual dose increases of methadone over a period of several weeks are usually not associated with any adverse effects. Dose increases do lead to the development of tolerance to the effects of opioids, however, so that the effects of injection of usual street doses of heroin are blocked or attenuated.

Finally, since methadone is chemically different from heroin, it is possible to use urine toxicology testing during methadone maintenance to evaluate whether there is persistence or cessation of use of heroin or other illicit drugs. With heroin maintenance, it would be impossible to determine whether a patient has curtailed illicit heroin use.

METHADONE TREATMENT CONSIDERATIONS

How well does methadone treatment work? One of the most illustrative studies from the perspectives of both treatment outcome and public policy effects was conducted in Sweden in the 1970s (Gronbladh 1989). Thirty-four patients were randomly assigned to either methadone maintenance treatment or drug-free outpatient treatment. During the period of the study, drug-free outpatient treatment was the predominant approach used for heroin-dependent patients in Sweden, so that the results for the drug-free treatment group might be about as good as could possibly be expected.

The study was called to a halt after two years because the findings were so compelling: in the methadone group, twelve patients were abstinent from illicit drug use and were either working or in school, while five had continuing drug abuse problems. One of these five was in prison, and another had been discharged from treatment because of continuing sedative abuse. In the drug-free treatment group, only one patient was abstinent from illicit drug use. Two were in prison, two had died from drug-related causes, and twelve had continuing drug abuse problems, including three who had suffered severe medical complications related to drug abuse. Perhaps not surprising, given the history of treatments for heroin addiction, shortly after completion of this study the methadone program stopped admitting new patients because of political opposition to this form of treatment.

The effectiveness of methadone maintenance treatment has been extensively documented through randomized clinical trials, quasi-experimental studies, and program evaluations. The original studies conducted by Dole and Nyswander showed astonishingly good results in comparison to historical controls (Dole and Nyswander 1965). Typically, more than 90 percent of patients relapse to heroin use within one year following detoxification. Yet, after two years of methadone treatment, only 13 of the initial 128 patients enrolled had been discharged for drug abuse or antisocial behavior. Of the 107 patients remaining in treatment, 71 percent were steadily employed or in school, and none had relapsed to heroin use. More recently, one-year retention rates in methadone programs still average 50 percent or more, far exceeding retention rates for any other treatment approach. Large-scale follow-up studies (for example, Treatment Outcome Prospective Study and Drug Abuse Reporting Program) demonstrate substantial reductions in both illicit drug use and criminal activity following methadone maintenance treatment entry (Hubbard et al. 1989; Simpson and Sells 1990).

Natural social experiments provide additional evidence of the effectiveness of the treatment. Following closure of the only methadone program in one California city in 1976, 54 percent of patients terminated from the program became readdicted to heroin within two years. In comparison, 31 percent of similar patients from a methadone program in another county that remained in operation became readdicted to heroin during this period. Arrest rates and incarceration rates among patients affected by the program closure were double the rates in the comparison group (Anglin et al. 1989). As suggested by the results of the Swedish methadone study, methadone maintenance is also associated with a substantial reduction (about 75 percent) in the excess annual mortality rate experienced by heroin addicts. In a study conducted in Philadelphia in 1989–91, 3.5 percent of methadone maintained patients became infected with HIV during an eighteen-month period, while 22 percent of untreated heroin addicts became infected during the same period (Metzger et al. 1993).

Despite these extremely positive findings, however, there are a number of problems limiting the overall effectiveness of methadone maintenance treatment. First, consistent with the history of addiction treatment as reviewed by William White (1998), widespread implementation of methadone maintenance treatment has led to considerable program-to-program variability in results. In one study of six programs in the Northeast, rates of illicit drug use ranged from less than 10 percent to more than 60 percent (Ball and Ross 1991). Methadone dose, length of treatment, and program stability powerfully influenced outcome. Patients treated at higher methadone doses and for longer periods of time had substantially lower rates of illicit drug use than patients treated at lower doses or for shorter periods of time. Higher methadone doses appear to be more effective in reducing craving and blocking the effects of street heroin use, and the association between higher doses and improved outcome has been noted since the inception of methadone maintenance treatment. Despite compelling evidence regarding the importance of adequate dosage, however, in the late 1980s the majority of methadone programs in the United States were using inadequate doses (D'Aunno and Vaughn 1992).

Several studies have demonstrated the dose-dependent efficacy of methadone with regard to retention and decreased rates of illicit opioid use more rigorously, through random assignment and double blind study design (Strain et al. 1993; Schottenfeld et al. 1997). In some jurisdictions, methadone doses continue to be limited by regulations, and in some programs doses are limited by program philosophy (Rettig and Yarmolinsky 1995). Similarly, while many patients require prolonged periods to achieve sufficient stability to be able to discontinue methadone maintenance without relapsing, and others may require lifelong maintenance, regulations and program philosophies often dictate shorter, inadequate treatment duration.

Counseling is also an essential component of effective methadone maintenance treatment. McLellan and his colleagues (1993) in Philadelphia randomly assigned new entrants to methadone treatment to one of three levels of counseling: minimal services (monthly brief counseling), standard services (weekly counseling, including behavioral interventions contingent on urine test results), and enhanced services (weekly counseling and onsite medical, psychiatric, employment, and family services). All patients were maintained at comparable and adequate methadone doses. The results of the study are striking. Nearly 70 percent of patients assigned to minimal services required protective transfer to standard services because of unremitting illicit drug use or medical or psychiatric emergency, whereas only 41 percent of the standard services group and 19 percent of the enhanced services group met the criteria for protective transfer. Rates of continued illicit opioid and cocaine use also were significantly higher in the minimal services group than in either the standard or enhanced services groups. While only 22 percent of patients receiving minimal services achieved eight or more consecutive weeks of abstinence from illicit opioids during the twenty-four-week study period, over 90 percent of patients in the standard and enhanced services groups were abstinent for at least eight consecutive weeks.

Considering only those patients who completed the twenty-four-week study, patients in the minimal services group reduced their use of illicit drugs but did not improve in any other outcome, while patients in the standard and enhanced services groups showed improvements in alcohol, legal, family, and psychiatric problem measures in addition to reductions in illicit drug use. In general, there was a consistent gradient in outcome, with more intensive services associated with greater improvements (McLellan et al. 1993). Subsequent cost-effectiveness analyses suggest that standard services were the most cost-effective approach (Kraft et al. 1997).

Cocaine abuse and abuse of alcohol and other substances also have become significant problems in methadone treatment programs (Schottenfeld et al. 1997). While most studies suggest that abuse of other substances is a problem for patients prior to entering methadone treatment and does not increase as a result of entry into methadone maintenance treatment, non-opioid substance abuse does interfere with rehabilitation (Condelli 1991). Rates of cocaine abuse among methadone patients range from 15 percent to 40 percent or even higher. Cocaine abuse is particularly problematic, since it is associated with an increased risk for HIV infection; increased family, medical, and vocational problems; and a continued focus on drug-related social interactions and criminal activity (Kolar et al. 1990).

There is considerable controversy about the policy implications of various responses to continued cocaine abuse during methadone treatment, ranging from "Don't ask/Don't tell" to discharging patients from treatment if they remain cocaine-dependent (Caulkins and Satel 1999). If there is insufficient treatment capacity, discharging of patients who are responding poorly or not at all may make room for new patients who can benefit from treatment. In some areas, however, there are no waiting lists, so that there is no need to discharge one patient to admit another. In this situation, the policy implications are less clear. Individual patients may benefit marginally from remaining on methadone treatment by reducing their heroin use even while continuing to use cocaine or to inject heroin less frequently.

Alternatively, continued and persistent use of cocaine or other illicit drugs, despite adequate methadone doses, intensive counseling, and psychiatric and other services, may be viewed as indicative of a poor response to the level of services available in the program. These patients remain at high risk of all of the adverse medical, personal, and social consequences of cocaine dependence. Consequently, they may benefit from referral to more intensive treatment, such as hospital or residential treatment, and continuation on methadone maintenance may only delay initiation of more appropriate and effective treatment. In addition, many patients benefit greatly from the setting of relatively firm limits in methadone treatment programs, and many patients with concurrent opioid and cocaine dependence are motivated to become abstinent in part because of administrative pressures on them to stop illicit drug use, including the possibility of being discharged from treatment for continued illicit drug use. Discharging patients who continue persistent drug use and are not benefiting or only partially benefiting from methadone treatment also conserves public resources even if there are no waiting lists for treatment entry.

Fewer than 20 percent of the estimated 600,000–750,000 heroin addicts in the United States are enrolled in methadone treatment, and probably fewer than half of all heroin addicts have ever received methadone maintenance treatment (NIH Consensus Panel 1998). A major rationale for proposing heroin maintenance programs is that this strategy may be more attractive than methadone maintenance for the large number of untreated heroin addicts. The limited reach of methadone maintenance treatment, its lack of market penetration, is a major problem, yet it is not at all clear that heroin maintenance is the only or the best solution, or that it is a solution at all. Prior to calling for initiation of heroin maintenance even as a trial program, we ought first to consider the reasons behind such low market penetration by methadone maintenance, and the range of options that could be employed to increase the reach of heroin addiction treatment.

One of the major factors limiting heroin addicts' participation in maintenance treatment has been inadequate funding and insurance coverage. In many regions, funding has simply not been available to increase treatment capacity, and long waiting lists to enter treatment deter many addicts from even trying. Over the past several years, Medicaid coverage for methadone treatment has allowed expansion of treatment capacity in Connecticut, and the number of patients enrolled in methadone programs in New Haven has more than doubled. Recent implementation of a rapid-intake unit, which enables addicts to begin methadone treatment within two or three days of initial contact, has more than doubled again the number of admissions to the programs. Currently, more than half of the patients admitted to our programs have never before been in methadone treatment.

These findings suggest that expanding methadone maintenance treatment capacity and facilitating rapid admission into programs can substantially reduce the number of untreated heroin addicts. Because treatment capacity has been limited, most programs have not undertaken aggressive outreach or marketing activities. We have successfully used mobile medical vans, neighborhood outreach workers, and cooperation with needle exchange programs to contact untreated heroin addicts and encourage them to enter treatment. More outreach might substantially reduce the number of untreated addicts.

Surprisingly little market research has been devoted to understanding the barriers to treatment entry. In addition to the problems of capacity and speed of admission, barriers include limited patient and community acceptance of methadone, the stigma associated with treatment in a maintenance clinic, and the loss of privacy attendant on using a drug abuse clinic. Of course the lack of availability in many areas of the country—it's still not permitted in many states (for example, Vermont)—is another major barrier. Some addicts may avoid methadone because of concerns that withdrawal will be even more difficult than it is from heroin. Myths about methadone, including the belief that methadone rots your bones, also remain prevalent among heroin addicts and discourage treatment entry. The need for daily dosing, combined with restrictions on take-home doses because of concerns about possible diversion, impose additional burdens on programs and on patients, who must come to the clinic daily. Addicts may also object to the counseling and other requirements of methadone programs. If this is the case, finding the optimal balance between encouraging treatment entry (at the expense of treatment efficacy) and encouraging efficacy (at the expense of discouraging program utilization) will be critical. The results of the Amsterdam low-threshold methadone program may provide some guidance about how best to balance these concerns (Hartgers et al. 1992).

Beginning in the early 1980s, Amsterdam developed a low-threshold methadone maintenance program that was designed to reduce the risk of hepatitis transmission and encourage heroin addicts to utilize medical and drug treatment services. Mobile methadone programs located on specially equipped buses followed fixed daily routes in the city, facilitating patient access and reducing problems of congestion, loitering, and neighborhood opposition attendant on locating programs permanently in one facility. Low-threshold programs allowed rapid entry into treatment and did not prohibit or discharge patients for illicit drug use. Daily methadone doses averaged approximately 35 mg, and no efforts were made to increase the doses in response to continued heroin use, out of concern that this would discourage addicts from seeking or remaining in treatment.

By all accounts, the program was remarkably effective in gaining access to heroin addicts. Approximately 65–70 percent of the heroin addicts in

Amsterdam were treated in the methadone program every year, and it has been estimated that 70–90 percent had at least some contact with the programs. Despite increasing access to treatment services, however, the program was not effective in reducing HIV transmission. Long-term regular participants in the program had more than twice the rate of HIV infection of short-term or irregular participants in the program, even controlling for other differences among the two groups. There was no evidence that daily participation in the program provided any protection against HIV seroconversion, and there was no reduction in the prevalence of injection drug use following program entry. Nearly one-third of addicts who entered the program prior to 1981 became infected with HIV over the following six to eight years. These results stand in stark contrast to the protective effects of methadone maintenance treatment found in the Philadelphia study (Metzger et al. 1993).

IMPROVING MAINTENANCE TREATMENT

Developing alternatives to methadone for opioid agonist maintenance treatment is one promising avenue for expanding the reach and attractiveness of treatment. Some medications may be more attractive to heroin addicts or may have other advantages that would facilitate their use in novel settings, such as primary care clinics or physicians' offices. Levo-acetyl alpha methadol (LAAM) was approved by the FDA in 1993 as the first alternative to methadone for maintenance treatment of opioid dependence (Glanz 1997). Like methadone, LAAM acts as a pure agonist at the mu receptor, so that it shares many of the problems associated with methadone, including possibility of overdose and difficulty of withdrawal. Because LAAM, with its active metabolites, is even longer-acting than methadone, however, it can be administered on a thrice-weekly dosing schedule, which permits reduced clinic attendance, obviates some of the need for take-home bottles (and the attendant problems of diversion for street use), and reduces dispensing costs.

A third medication, buprenorphine, is also under investigation for maintenance treatment and appears likely to gain FDA approval soon. Buprenorphine is a high-affinity partial agonist at the mu receptor, that is, although it binds even more tightly to the receptor than heroin or methadone, it only partially activates the receptor. One of the interesting issues in the history of research on buprenorphine, which resonates with episodes in the history of the early heroin studies, is that it was initially thought that there was no withdrawal associated with abrupt buprenorphine discontinuation because buprenorphine has both agonist and antagonist effects. More recently, withdrawal symptoms have been observed, especially in patients maintained at higher doses (Fudala et al. 1990). The apparent lack of withdrawal noted earlier most likely resulted from the very slow dissociation of buprenorphine from the mu opiate receptor. Because of this slow dissociation, buprenorphine, like LAAM, need not be administered as frequently as methadone. It has recently been shown that a thrice-weekly dosage is as effective as daily administration (Schottenfeld et al. 1998), and Ed Johnson and his colleagues have shown that thrice-weekly buprenorphine is comparable to LAAM and only slightly less efficacious than methadone with regard to reductions in illicit opioid use (Johnson et al. 2000). Because of its pharmacologic properties, the risk of overdose and abuse liability associated with buprenorphine is considerably less than that for either methadone or LAAM. The low abuse liability of buprenorphine, especially in the form of a tablet that incorporates a quantity of the opioid antagonist naloxone to discourage injection use, may permit scheduling buprenorphine for use outside of traditional maintenance clinics.

This development would dovetail nicely with a second strategy to expand the reach of agonist maintenance treatment—utilization of primary care and medical office settings. Utilizing primary care settings to provide maintenance treatment would be a relatively easy way of expanding the availability of drug treatment and improving access to treatment for individuals already utilizing primary care settings. Primary care sites are widely dispersed throughout the United States, including cities that do not have traditional agonist maintenance programs. Many out-of-treatment addicts use primary care settings for treatment of medical complications of opiate dependence. Maintenance treatment within the primary care setting may decrease the likelihood of the person in recovery coming in contact with an active drug user, as occurs at treatment centers. Primary care centers are also less stigmatizing for patients, are easier to access, and provide greater privacy.

In concluding, I would like to make a modest counterproposal to either implementation of heroin maintenance or elimination of methadone maintenance. I suggest that we first implement a series of policies and programs to increase the number of heroin addicts enrolled in current drug abuse treatments. This approach presumably would utilize a combination of capacity expansion, modifications of programs so as to make them more convenient and appealing to heroin addicts (for example, expanded hours, mobile or neighborhood locations, and so forth), concerted outreach, development of primary care programs, and coordination with criminal justice system initiatives. We could then track the impact of aggressively marketed expanded treatment on important social indicators, such as rates of theft, burglary, and robbery. New Haven would be an ideal city in which to try this approach: it's small enough to provide the opportunity to try these proposals and succeed on a relatively modest budget.

If this trial is successful, the protocols developed could be used in other regions. If some number of heroin addicts chose to remain untreated under such an improved system, we would then be in a position to evaluate whether offering heroin maintenance, or any other new treatment, leads that group to enter treatment and whether these most-difficult-to-reach patients would benefit from such a program. Of course, this full-capacity and multimodality treatment system also would serve as an ideal laboratory for evaluating competing policy options, such as determining the optimal balance between treatment efficacy, which relies on relatively highly structured programs, and treatment reach, which improves with less structured options. Finally, this planned natural experiment would provide an ideal opportunity to evaluate the broader social benefits of expanding treatment capacity and reach—that is, the impact on rates of criminal activity, child abuse or neglect, unemployment, and public assistance utilization.

Mindful of the history of heroin addiction treatment in the United States, I wonder whether this proposal doesn't seem similar to the development and rapid expansion of multimodality treatments for heroin addiction pioneered in the 1960s in Chicago, Washington, D.C., New Haven, and other cities, which led to dramatic reductions in drug-related crime and improved the health of addicts. At times, we could do worse than to repeat the accomplishments of our forebears.

REFERENCES

Anglin, M. D., G. R. Speckart, M. W. Booth, and T. M. Ryan. 1989. "Consequences and Costs of Shutting Off Methadone." *Addictive Behaviors* 14:307–26.

Ball, J. C., and A. Ross. 1991. *The Effectiveness of Methadone Maintenance Treatment.* New York: Springer-Verlag.

Caulkins, J. P., and S. L. Satel. 1999. "Methadone Patients Should Not Be Allowed to Persist in Cocaine Use." *Drug Policy Analysis Bulletin* 6:1–5.

Condelli, W. S., J. A. Fairbank, M. L. Dennis, and J. V. Rachal. 1991. "Cocaine Use by Clients in Methadone Programs: Significance, Scope, and Behavioral Interventions." *Journal of Substance Abuse Treatment* 8:203–12.

Cornish, J. W., D. Metzger, G. E. Woody, D. Wilson, A. T. McLellan, B. Vandergrift, and C. P. O'Brien. 1997. "Naltrexone Pharmacotherapy for Opioid Dependent Federal Probationers." *Journal of Substance Abuse Treatment* 14:529–34.

D'Aunno, T., and T. E. Vaughn. 1992. "Variations in Methadone Treatment Practices." *JAMA* 267:253–58.

Dole, V. P. 1988. "Implications of Methadone Maintenance for Theories of Narcotic Addiction." *JAMA* 260: 3025–29.

Dole V. P., and M. Nyswander. 1965. "A Medical Treatment for Diacetylmorphine (Heroin) Addiction." *JAMA* 193:80–84.

Fudala, J. P., J. H. Jaffe, E. M. Dax, and R. E. Johnson. 1990. "Use of Buprenorphine in the Treatment of Opioid Addiction. II.: Physiologic and Behavioral Effects of Daily and Alternate-Day Administration and Abrupt Withdrawal." *Clinical Pharmacology and Therapeutics* 35:89–92.

194   TREATMENT OPTIONS

Ginzburg, H. M. 1989. *Drug Abuse Treatment: National Study of Effectiveness*. Chapel Hill: University of North Carolina Press.

Glanz, M., S. Klawansky, W. McAuliffe, and T. Chalmers. 1997. "Methadone vs. L-alpha-acetylmethadol (LAAM) in the Treatment of Opiate Addiction." *American Journal on Addictions* 6:339–49.

Gronbladh, L., and L. Gunne. 1989. "Methadone-Assisted Rehabilitation of Swedish Heroin Addicts." *Drug and Alcohol Dependence* 24:31–37.

Hartgers, C., A. van den Hoek, P. Krijnen, and R. A. Coutinho. 1992. "HIV Prevalence and Risk Behavior Among Injecting Drug Users Who Participate in 'Low-Threshold' Methadone Program in Amsterdam." *American Journal of Public Health* 82:547–51.

Hubbard, R. L., M. E. Marsden, J. V. Rachal, H. J. Harwood, E. R. Cavanaugh, and

Johnson, R. E., M. A. Chutuape, E. C. Strain, S. L. Walsh, M. L. Stitzer, and G. E. Bigelow. 2000. "A Comparison of Levomethadyl Acetate, Buprenorphine, and Methadone for Opioid Dependence." *New England Journal of Medicine* 343:1290–97.

Kolar, A. F., B. S. Brown, W. W. Weddington, and J. C. Ball. 1990. "A Treatment Crisis: Cocaine Use by Clients in Methadone Programs." *Journal of Substance Abuse Treatment* 7:101–07.

Kraft, M. K., A. B. Rothbard, T. R. Hadley, A. T. McLellan, and D. A. Asch. 1997. "Are Supplementary Services Provided During Methadone Maintenance Really Cost- Effective?" *American Journal of Psychiatry* 154:1214–19.

McLellan, A. T., I. O. Arndt, D. S. Metzger, G. E. Woody, and C. P. O'Brien. 1993. "The Effects of Psychosocial Services in Substance Abuse Treatment." *JAMA* 269: 1943–59.

Metzger, D. S., G. E. Woody, A. T. McLellan, C. P. O'Brien, P. Druley, H. Navaline, D. DePhilippis, P. Stolley, and E. Abrutyn. 1993. "Human Immunodeficiency Virus Seroconversion Among Intravenous Drug Users In-and-Out-of-Treatment: An 18-Month Prospective Follow-up." *Journal of Acquired Immunodeficiency Syndromes* 6:1049–56.

Meyer, R. E., and S. M. Mirin, eds. 1979. *The Heroin Stimulus*. New York: Plenum Press.

Nestler, E. J. 1992. "Molecular Mechanisms of Drug Addiction." *Journal of Neuroscience* 12:2439–50.

NIH Consensus Panel. 1998. "Consensus Development Panel on Effective Medical Treatment of Opiate Addiction." *JAMA* 280:1936–43.

Novick, D. M., M. Ochshorn, V. Ghali, T. S. Croxson, W. D. Mercer, N. Chiorazzi, and M. J. Kreek. 1989. "Natural Killer-Cell Activity and Lymphocyte Subsets in Parental Heroin Abusers and Long-term Methadone Maintenance Patients." *Journal of Pharmacology and Experimental Therapies* 250:606–10.

O'Malley, S. S., A. J. Jaffe, G. Chang, R. S. Schottenfeld, R. E. Meyer, and B. J. Rounsaville. 1992. "Naltrexone and Coping Skills Therapy for Alcohol Dependence: A Controlled Study." *Archives of General Psychiatry* 49:881–87.

Petitjean, S., and D. Ladewig. 2000. "Effects of Intravenous Heroin on Psychomotor and Cognitive Functioning in Humans." *College on Problems of Drug Dependence 2000 Annual Meeting Abstracts*.

Rettig, R. A., and A. Yarmolinsky, eds. 1995. *Federal Regulations of Methadone Treatment*. Washington, D.C.: Institute of Medicine, National Academy Press.

Rounsaville, B. J. 1995. "Can Psychotherapy Rescue Naltrexone Treatment of Opioid Addiction?" *NIDA Research Monograph* 150:37–52.

Schottenfeld, R. S., J. R. Pakes, and T. R. Kosten. 1998. "Prognostic Factors in Buprenorphine- vs. Methadone-maintained Patients." *Journal of Nervous and Mental Disease* 186:35–43.

Schottenfeld, R. S., J. P. Pakes, A. Oliveto, D. Ziedonis, and T. R. Kosten. 1997. "Buprenorphine vs. Methadone Maintenance Treatment for Concurrent Opioid Dependence and Cocaine Use." *Archives of General Psychiatry* 54:713–20.

Simpson, D. D., and S. G. Sells, eds. 1990. *Opioid Addiction and Treatment: A 12-Year Follow-up*. Malabar: Robert E. Krieger.

Strain, E. C., M. L. Stitzer, I. A. Liebson, and G. E. Bigelow. 1993. "Dose-response Effects of Methadone in the Treatment of Opioid Dependence." *Annals of Internal Medicine* 119:23–27.

White, W. L. 1998. *Slaying the Dragon: The History of Addiction Treatment and Recovery in America*. Bloomington, Ill.: Chestnut Health Systems/Lighthouse Institute.

Part V

Political and Cultural Complications

12

From British India to the Taliban: Lessons from the History of the Heroin Market

Kathryn Meyer

In September 1997 Pino Arlacchi became head of the United Nations International Drug Control Program. He had impressive credentials for an international drug czar: he began his career as a professor of sociology. His excellent books about the Italian Mafia had brought him recognition as a leading expert on organized crime. Unlike most scholars, he had put his knowledge into action; he had joined the Italian Parliament and had led an attack against the same criminals whose organization he had researched. By all reports he was successful in his efforts to bring the Sicilian Mafia under control (see *Financial Times* [London], July 17, 1997; *New York Times*, June 23, 1997).

From his new position Arlacchi announced the beginning of a ten-year plan to eradicate narcotics worldwide. He then opened discussions with the Taliban, the revolutionary Islamic group in control of war-torn Afghanistan, a major poppy-growing area supplying today's heroin market. To his surprise, the Taliban leadership indicated a willingness to work with the United Nations. Thus, in mid-November 1997 Arlacchi went to Afghanistan to discuss concrete plans to provide funds for irrigation projects and a textile factory, all to be built in a key opium growing area. His trip provided the Taliban with an opportunity to enhance their international image, tarnished by numerous accounts of religious intolerance and poor treatment of women. Because he was criticized in some circles for making compromises with repressive regimes, Arlacchi was careful to point out the positive contributions U.N.

aid would make, including plans for a wool-weaving plant that would employ women (*New York Times*, October 25, 1997, November 14, 1997; Associated Press, November 27, 1997, Lexis/Nexis).

Arlacchi's Afghan trip was the forerunner of a larger global plan to eliminate drug crops through "alternative development." "We would propose an alternative way of life," he told Christopher Wren of the *New York Times*. "They can be rich peasants if they grow opium, but they can die if they don't have roads and hospitals." His plan was not all carrot and no stick, however; it called for enforcement as well. He summarized it as "alternative development, eradication and law enforcement." The program was endorsed by the Clinton administration and General Barry McCaffrey, the reigning U.S. drug czar, applauded Arlacchi's "focused, high-energy leadership" (*New York Times*, November 25, 1997, December 3, 1997, June 7, 1998).

Yet, in spite of the public professions of compliance by the Taliban, poppy production in Taliban-controlled areas continued. The 1998 harvest was about as large as that of the previous year. In response, Arlacchi told nations contributing aid to Afghanistan that he was prepared to use the earmarked money for border patrols rather than development. Noorullah Zadran, a Taliban spokesman, replied, "God knows we tried. There is a difference in cultures. There is a different perception" (*New York Times*, July 17, 1998). Afghanistan is indeed a place with a distinct culture; however, both Zadran and Arlacchi were wrong if they thought that this made the Afghani situation unique. These two men and their respective organizations fit into a pattern that has been repeated throughout the first hundred years of the illicit heroin market.

Over the course of the twentieth century the major areas of both poppy production and heroin consumption shifted. Before the Communist revolution of 1949, China was the world's major consumer; since the early 1950s the United States and Europe have assumed that role. Early in the nineteenth century heroin made only small inroads onto a market dominated by smoking opium; today it is the most visible illicit opiate available. The opiate market has been defined by the difficulties of delivering a desirable product through an increasing network of international regulations. These laws, rather than ending the traffic, became part of the risk of engaging in a highly profitable trade. Looking at the development of this enterprise may provide some lessons for Mr. Arlacchi.

POPPIES, OPIUM, AND ASIA

The earliest international sanctions against narcotics came in China, only eight years after the invention of heroin. Opium use and cultivation had been legal in that country from 1858 to 1906. Although, at that time, opium smoking was considered to be a Chinese vice, the poppy plant was not native to Asia, nor was the fifty-year-long legality of the drug a policy willingly adopted by the Chinese government. Legalization was accepted by a weakened Chinese government after China's bold attempts to force British smugglers to withdraw from its shores had enmeshed it in a losing struggle with the British navy. The opium problem was a nagging reminder of a larger attack on the authority of the Chinese state by foreigners.

The best opium came from British India. In 1905, when British diplomats suggested the possibility of opium restriction, the Chinese government responded positively. Statesmen representing the emperor knew they required British participation for any domestic program to prove effective. In 1906 China's opium eradication began with edicts against the cultivation and use of opium in China. This was followed by a British measure restricting exports of opium from India to China. The Qing (Ch'ing or Manchu) dynasty government that began this ambitious project had only five years left in its 270-year reign. On its last legs, it faced general public disorder, economic decline, and increasing foreign encroachment. Yet, as government officials began closing down opium dens and plowing-under poppy fields, they were met with public enthusiasm and surprising success (see *North China Herald* February 8, 1907, April 26, 1907; Hosie 1914, v. 2, 191; and Riens 1991).

In 1911 the Qing dynasty was overthrown and in 1912 a new republic was declared. Best known in the West for its figurehead leader Sun Yat-sen and his Guomindang, or Nationalist party, the republic was in its early years dominated by the military strongman Yuan Shikai, who immediately began chipping away at the constitution and attacking those who opposed him. Yet, in spite of political conflicts between Sun's democratic ideals and Yuan's authoritarian ambitions, opium reform moved forward after only a short pause. Part of the motivation behind the success was the determination of Chinese patriots to rid their country of a problem that they saw as debilitating to the nation, a plague brought in by foreigners (*North China Herald*, October 12, 1912; Jordan to Grey, March 5, 1912, FO 10168/12644, and Jordan to Grey, January 22, 1913, FO 10481/6308, in Great Britain, Foreign Office 1974).

Narcotics regulation began in this climate of political breakdown, promoted by people with larger political agendas. Suppliers and addicts adapted to the new conditions as best they could. Legitimate opium merchants shifted their business arrangements. Some wealthy addicts bought up the last of the legal supply, while many others tried cures. There were different remedies, however. By 1917, when these first reform campaigns collapsed, "white drugs," including heroin, appeared in China and were advanced as cheaper, more easily transportable alternatives to opium and sometimes as a cure for the opium habit. Thus, the introduction of heroin into the Chinese opiate market was dictated by the necessity of circumventing legal barriers. David

Courtwright notes that the same process occurred in America after passage of the Smoking Opium Exclusion Act of 1909 (Courtwright 1982, 83).

THE CHINESE OPIUM BUSINESS TAKES A NEW DIRECTION

The Taliban assured Mr. Arlacchi that the use of intoxicants is contrary to Islam and that, therefore, their own beliefs required them to end Afghani trafficking. At the same time they obviously relied on opium profits to continue their war efforts, making them appear to be hypocrites of the first order. In fact, the Taliban were responding to a complex political scenario strikingly similar to an episode that occurred in China only ten years after the first opium bans went into effect. The smuggling case associated with the Righteous Yunnan Uprising of 1916 marked the breakdown of the first successful opium reform and demonstrates how illicit delivery systems can become political tools.

One of the most surprising victories during the ten-year opium reform in China came from Yunnan province. Yunnan shares a border with both Burma and what was then French Indochina, just north of the area known today as the Golden Triangle. Because it had been established as a commercial poppy growing area during the fifty years in which opium was legal, it came as a surprise to reformers when reports appeared in 1909 that Yunnan was on the road to opium eradication. Local officials were thorough, even giving thought to what we now call crop substitution. Change proceeded despite the obstacle that while opium was moved easily over the rugged Yunnan terrain, rice did not have such an agreeable portability. And when a bumper crop of rice glutted the local market in 1914, officials recommended producing rice wine, to help peasants stave off the temptation to resort to their opium standby (Hosie 1914, v. 2, app. 2; Butler to Grey, February 9, 1910, FO 9392/9773, Great Britain, Foreign Office 1974; *North China Herald*, October 10, 1914).

Then, in 1916 Yunnan became the base of operations for a group of patriotic soldiers who opposed Yuan Shikai. For two years after the 1911 revolution Chinese politicians had tried to create a constitution and convene a parliament. Yuan, however, dismantled those attempts and became more of a dictator. With each step toward authoritarian rule, Yuan alienated more of his supporters. The last straw came in 1915, when he cast aside all pretense of republicanism and proclaimed himself Emperor of China. Yuan's power came from his control of the Chinese army. Many of his officers had supported the revolt against the previous imperial house. The absurdity of Yuan's imperial ambitions made these once-loyal supporters back away from him. Cai E was one of these officers. From his stronghold in Yunnan province he formed the Protect the Nation Army and led a revolt against Yuan (Yu 1966 [1917]; Zhang 1986).

Cai E was from a gentry family. He had given up scholarship and trained for a military career because he feared the weakness of China in the modern world. He was ascetic and dedicated to the republican cause. In December 1915 the National Protection Army began an armed revolt, as other officers declared themselves independent of Yuan's erstwhile empire. Yunnan began to attract patriots from all over China, including some members of Sun Yat-sen's Guomindang. In the face of such overwhelming opposition, Yuan Shikai gave up his imperial scheme in May 1916. He died in June 1916 (Ch'en 1972).

This military exercise, though brief, had been expensive. During the struggle with Yuan the Yunnan patriots remained in contact with sympathetic groups throughout China, including the Guomindang in Shanghai, which sent much-needed funds. The Guomindang, in turn, relied on some of the more unsavory characters in Shanghai for fund-raising. Shanghai Municipal Police blotters were filled with complaints about the strong-arm tactics used to raise money for the revolt. Also during this period Yunnan opium began flowing once again onto the China market (Shanghai Municipal Police, 1916).

The short revolt and Yuan's subsequent death left a power vacuum in China. Cai E's generals, hailed as heroes, began to plan a greater national role for themselves in the aftermath of victory. In the summer of 1916 the many factions that had united against Yuan came together in Beijing to plan China's political future. Yunnan sent a delegation that left the province on June 23. The generals traveled by train south through French Indochina to Haiphong, where they caught a ship to Shanghai (map 12.1).

The Yunnan party hoped to use the visibility they had gained during the war to move into national prominence. To this end, they determined to establish a partisan newspaper and publicity office in Shanghai. They were, however, short on funds, and so they turned to smuggling. Having acquired a supply of opium that had been confiscated by Yunnan police during the earlier poppy eradication campaigns, they loaded it into the trunks that would accompany them on their journey. They felt safe because a prominent member of the old Parliament accompanied them, but just to be sure, they packed opium in his trunks as well (Zhang 1986; Minguo Ribao [Republican Daily], August 9–23, 1916; Shi Bao [Eastern Times], August 9–23, 1916; North China Herald, August 9–23, 1916).

Shanghai was the best place from which to move opium onto the Chinese market. As the entrepôt to the Yangzi (Yangtze) River, it provided access to trade routes running through the country, making it the entrepreneurial center of China. Shanghai also had a significant foreign presence and had been

Map 12.1
Route Traveled by the Yunnan Patriots and Their Opium-Laden Baggage

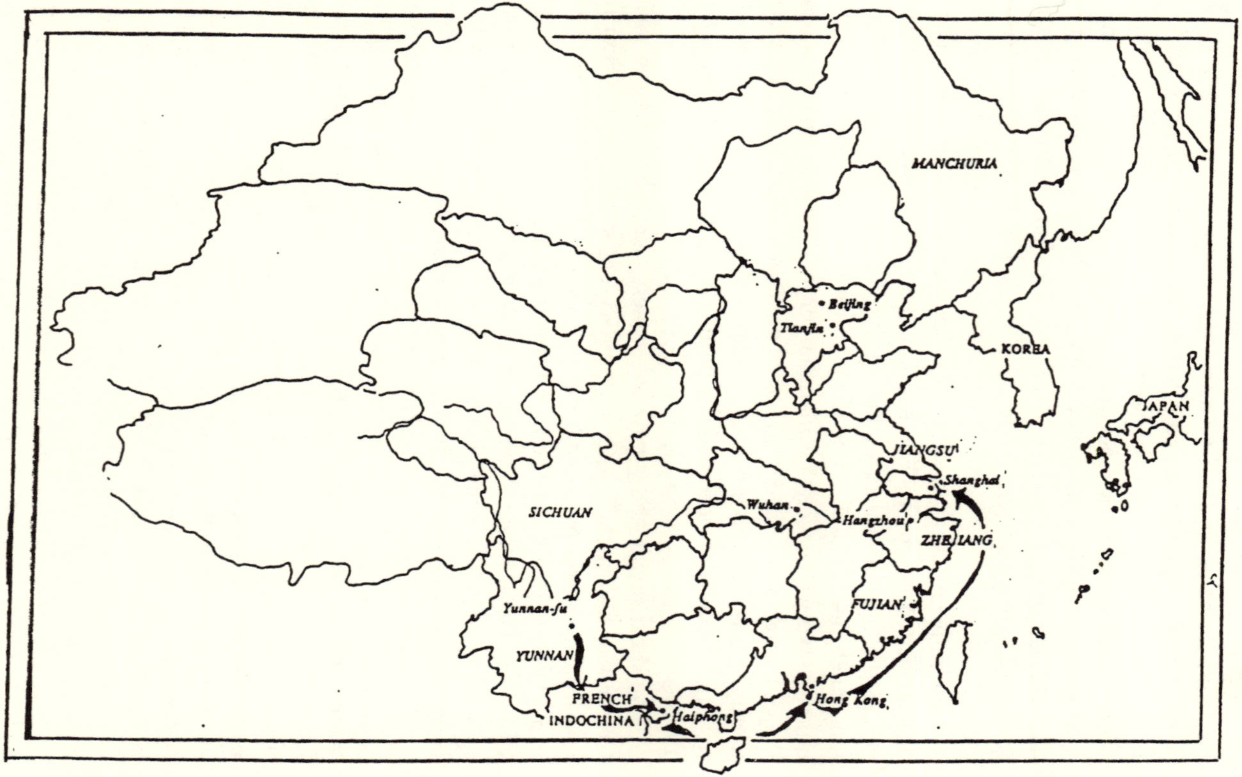

fragmented politically into a French concession; the International Settlement, where British and other foreign nationals lived; and a large, sprawling Chinese city. Each area had its own courts and police jurisdictions, making law enforcement difficult under the best of conditions (Zhang 1985).

The opium-laden trunks, sixty in all, easily cleared customs because the Yunnan generals had political connections. The men and their luggage then went to a Chinese inn in Shanghai's International Settlement. But the next evening international police raided the hotel and confiscated four opium-filled trunks. On the following day police traced an additional twenty trunks to the office of a prominent Chinese official, the same man who had signed the customs waiver. When the case reached its conclusion, three members of the Yunnan party were convicted of smuggling, and several Chinese officials were so badly compromised that their careers ended (*Minguo Ribao*, August 22, 1916).

Cai E was never implicated in the scandal, and he probably knew nothing about the opium scheme. During the campaigns he was a busy man and a sick one. While his subordinates traveled to Shanghai to further their careers, he went there separately, seeking medical attention. Cai's subordinates were more practical and ambitious men than he. Tang Jiyao, the second in command, was very much implicated in the opium scandal. After the fiasco in Shanghai, Tang returned to Yunnan, where he retreated from national politics, making the province into his personal power base. By the 1920s, it was once again a major opium-producing area.

The Yunnan case established a pattern that repeated itself throughout the century, even as heroin replaced opium. The source of opium was in an area with a population poor enough to profit from such labor-intensive endeavors as poppy cultivation and opium manufacture and smuggling. More important, the undertaking was protected by ambitious men willing to make short-term compromises for larger political goals. Putting ideals into practice takes revenue. Many of the Yunnan leaders were against opium because it tarnished the republic, yet the state of civil war made the situation too complex for them to entirely control. Can we call these men simple hypocrites, or was something more complicated going on?

The Yunnan uprising of 1916 solved none of China's problems; Yuan's collapse left a power vacuum that was filled by contending military strongmen, commonly called the warlords, most of whom followed the Yunnan pattern and relied on opium funds. These warlords have such a bad reputation that it is well to recall that the first armed military revolt was filled with promise and is still referred to as the Righteous Yunnan Uprising. In the 1920s and 1930s this Chinese civil war continued. It changed direction in 1927 when the Guomindang nationalists eclipsed the warlords and fought the

Chinese Communists, while facing a serious Japanese threat. Opium and, increasingly, heroin thrived in this atmosphere.

THE BEGINNINGS OF INTERNATIONAL REGULATION

Pino Arlacchi brought to his career a passionate dedication that transcended the mere filling of a job description. This animated enthusiasm is a requirement for anyone hoping to create successful international reforms. Certainly the man who played a pivotal role in the 1920s League of Nations anti-opium efforts was equally passionate. Sir Malcolm Delevingne did not invent the international regulatory system, but the force of his personality gave it direction.

International efforts to regulate narcotics traffic began in the first years of the twentieth century. The encouraging signs coming from the Chinese reform effort of 1906 coincided with American legislation to curb narcotics. In the same year that China promulgated its anti-opium edicts, the U.S. government passed the Pure Food and Drug Act, the first of its many prohibitionist laws. Americans also were instrumental in calling the first international narcotics conference, convened at Shanghai in 1909 to discuss the issue of opium smoking throughout East Asia. Follow-up conferences at The Hague in 1911–12, 1913, and 1914 resulted in more substantial agreements that became the basis for League of Nations initiatives (Musto 1973, 24–53; Taylor 1973, 47–122).

The results of these first steps toward international opium control made the Chinese drug market change rather than disappear. As supplies of both Indian and domestic opium shrank, the skyrocketing price of smoking opium induced many Chinese to satisfy their craving through heroin. More powerful than opium, it was sometimes injected with a hypodermic syringe but more often was smoked, just as opium had been. Other commodities appeared as well. Red Pills and Gold Pills—capsules containing morphine that had been introduced as cures for opium addiction—soon became popular as cheap opium substitutes. During the ten years of successful opium suppression, a market for refined opiates developed in China. After 1917, when smoking opium became plentiful in China again, heroin use continued, especially among the urban lower classes (Public Record Office, London [hereafter, PRO], "Memorandum Respecting the Opium Problem in the Far East," August 10, 1929, 17–18; "Smuggling Opium into China," *Times* [London], March 27, 1920; Ah Nan 1937).

At first, heroin was not manufactured in China. A few European, American, and Japanese pharmaceutical firms produced the entire world's supply. After World War I opium control measures expanded to address the additional problem of narcotic substitutes. In 1921 the League of Nations created the Advisory Committee on Traffic in Opium and Other Dangerous Drugs, more commonly known as the Opium Advisory Committee (OAC). Between 1925 and 1936 it produced systems to control narcotics at their source. One such arrangement was the creation in 1925 of a certificate system to track the international movement of narcotic drugs. The purpose of the agreement was to eliminate the excessive production of narcotic drugs, which resulted in diversion of a substantial quantity into the illicit traffic. In addition to formulating conventions, the OAC did valuable work in less visible ways. It gathered and shared information about the "hot spots" in the drug traffic, and it put political pressure on supply nations, albeit with varying degrees of success (Parssinen 1983, 144, 151; "Foreign Office Minutes 1920," PRO FO 371/5307/117–20; "Conference on the Restrictions of Opium," July 19, 1920, PRO FO 371/5307;107–08).

The idea for the OAC came from the British government, and specifically from Malcolm Delevingne, who, as Home Office Undersecretary, had responsibility for the drug traffic. Like Pino Arlacchi, he made elimination of narcotics his life's goal. He became the driving force behind the League's efforts. During the 1920s information that he received about the sources and movement of narcotics led him to criticize certain European governments and firms for what he considered to be opportunism in finding and using loopholes in international regulations. An instance of this was his censure of the Swiss government's tolerance for the way Hoffmann La Roche slipped around the irregular European laws. This attitude, he said, demonstrated that they "do not take into account the character of the proceedings of the firm from a moral point of view" ("Memorandum Respecting Traffic in Opium," 1920, PRO FO 371/5308/233, 238–41; M. Delevingne to Foreign Office, February 27, 1926, PRO FO 371/11713/156). These efforts had their effect, although not entirely along the lines that Sir Malcolm had envisioned.

A CRISIS IN HEROIN SUPPLY

As a result of the efforts of Delevingne and the OAC, and despite footdragging by certain governments, the situation changed rapidly in Europe by the late 1920s. Enactment of the certificate system, universal enforcement of strictures against trafficking in western Europe by 1930, and the curtailment of production in European factories by 1932 had reduced legitimate opiate production to less than half of what it had been in 1928–29. This crisis of supply forced a restructuring of the entire industry.

One man whose career demonstrates the changes taking place in Europe is Elie Eliopoulos, a Greek national operating out of Paris. From 1928 to 1931 he sold morphine and heroin to Tianjin, China. He began his career just as it was becoming difficult for illicit traders to make legal purchases of European narcotics. British and American factories were closed to them, and Swiss and German manufacturers were beginning to feel government pressure. However, a few French factories continued to supply the market. Eliopoulos established connections with two of these—the Comptoir des Alcaloides and the Société Industrielle de Chimie Organique. In 1930, when the French government passed stronger legislation, restricting narcotics trading licenses to only fifteen or sixteen reputable firms, Eliopoulos adapted. He turned to Istanbul, where his old suppliers opened a factory called ETKIM (Eliopolous 1932; Moses 1933).

Eliopoulos needed political protection after January 1929, when the French laws took effect. Early in his career he had struck a bargain with an Inspector Martin of the Paris Prefecture of Police, who supplied protection in return for money. Eliopoulos at first paid Martin 5,000 francs per month; this amount doubled as the business flourished. Eliopoulos could afford even this higher business expense, for morphine and heroin purchased in Europe for £40 or less per kilo could be sold in Tianjin at £70 or more per kilo. Monthly receipts of £21,000 yielded a gross profit of about £9,000 on the Tianjin business alone. From Eliopoulos's perspective, protection was a manageable business expense. Martin protected Eliopolous until a Surete investigation in 1931 exposed Eliopoulos and made the situation untenable (Eliopoulos 1932).

Eliopoulos's trade with China was not his only narcotics business. Contrary to his profession, "by the memory of my father and all else that is holy," that he never sold drugs to America, he was a regular supplier of Jacob Polakiewitz, aka Jack Paull, then the largest exporter of narcotics to the United States (Eliopolous 1932; Moses 1933). Until the 1950s, however, this American market remained secondary to China.

Eliopoulos flourished during a period of crisis and transition in the illicit narcotics industry. At the end of his four-year career he described important changes taking place in the world market. As restrictive measures in France, Germany, and Turkey made it difficult to divert large quantities of narcotic drugs from European pharmaceutical houses, Asian traffickers had begun to use Chinese opium to manufacture their own narcotic drugs (Eliopoulos 1932, 16–17). It would be Chinese gangsters and Japanese adventurers who would actively develop the heroin market in the 1930s.

BLACK INTO WHITE

After ten years of successful opium reform in China, smoking opium returned to the market, but now it was supplied by smugglers and the price was considerably higher. Poorer addicts, who turned to morphine and heroin, accounted for the demand that Elie Eliopoulos supplied in the 1920s. As Eliopoulos himself observed, however, by the early 1930s, Asian chemists were learning the secret of turning black (opium) into white (morphine and heroin). And they had developed a better delivery system.

During the years in which Eliopoulos and other Europeans sold heroin to China, the Green Gang of Shanghai rationalized the opium distribution network by perfecting the kind of political connections the Yunnan opium group had tried to create. The Green Gang was well placed to step into the business. It had grown with the port, feeding on protection, gambling, labor racketeering, and prostitution. The gang controlled the wharves of Shanghai, an advantage for smuggling. It was a tip from a Green Gang member to the Shanghai police that had ruined the plans of the Yunnan group, whose biggest mistake was encroaching on someone else's territory (Zhang 1986).

The introduction of opium profits after the breakdown of reform made the 1910s contentious, as Green Gang factions fought over the lucrative trade. Only in the 1920s did three men known as the Three Big Shots—Huang Jinrong, Zhang Xiaolin, and Du Yuesheng—put together what would become in the 1930s a financial empire including both illicit and legitimate enterprises. They would create the kind of syndicate that their American contemporary Al Capone only briefly visualized before his collapse. Huang Jinrong brought with him to this enterprise his Shanghai police connections and Zhang Xiaolin, his influential friends in the military.

Du Yuesheng, the kingpin of the Green Gang, is as famous to the Chinese as Al Capone is to Americans. Du was able to expand his smuggling empire through building on political connections. His ultimate triumph came in 1927, when the Green Gang helped Chiang Kai-shek purge the Guomindang party of Chinese Communist members in a bloody massacre known as the white terror (Isaacs 1951, 143–85; Marshall 1977, 29–35). After this initial event, Du's opium money contributed to the Nationalist war chest. In return, Du was able to work in Shanghai with relative freedom from police harassment (Xiao 1996).

Du was a diplomat. He ended the violent conflicts that marked the early days of the illicit Chinese opium market through negotiation as much as through force. From 1920 on, he made peace with every military strongman in the Chinese civil war who ventured into or around Shanghai by negotiating agreements that could be mutually profitable. These early deals employed the kind of pure graft exchanged between Eliopolous and his Inspector Martin. When Du brokered a deal with Chiang Kai-shek, it was made on a pattern already established. Yet Chiang was not an ordinary warlord. He had a vision of national unity that was frustrated by the continuing Communist resistance (Martin 1996, 51–109; Mei and Shao 1987, 50–69).

Scholars have been both kind to and critical of Chiang Kai-shek. He has been praised by some as a nationalist hero and reviled by others as a narrow-minded bully. Those who attack him are quick to point out his alliance with

Du; those who honor him respond that Du used his gang to work against the Japanese army during World War II. The truth of the situation is not as simple as either side maintains. Chiang Kai-shek was no friend of the narcotics traffic. He was an abstemious man who thrived under military discipline. But, like the Taliban, he faced a political reality so complex and expensive that his attitudes about drug regulation were easily compromised. In the 1930s he faced both internal conflict and foreign invasion. He needed money, and he needed information.

One way of appreciating the revenue-generating power of opium at that time is to follow the change in its cost along the Yangzi River from Chongqing, deep in the opium-growing region of Sichuan, to Shanghai, on the coast. In Chongqing the cost of prepared opium was $1.50 per ounce; in Yichang it cost $2.00; in Hankou, $2.80; and in Shanghai, $4.50.[1] These price increases came from taxation. In 1932 the American consul, Walter A. Adams, conservatively estimated the total revenue produced by the Chinese opium traffic at $300 million per year. Over the decade of the 1930s, the nationalist government initiated opium monopoly schemes, which served to bring the traffic under government control. The profits went into the Agricultural Bank of China, where they funded intelligence operations (Stilwell 1935, 15; Adams 1934; Xiao 1996, v. 20, 609–17).

Du benefited from his alliance with Chiang Kai-shek. Yet there were times when his ambitions clashed with Chiang's sensibilities or with the plans of others also backed by Chiang. One example occurred in 1932, as Du was expanding into morphine and heroin manufacturing. Chiang gave Du a quantity of confiscated opium to make into medical morphine. Du created a processing plant to make the morphine, but he also secretly continued to operate the facility to make illicit heroin from opium that he received from another source. When Chiang learned of the extended operation, he sent police to raid the factory. It took several weeks of negotiation for Du to get himself back in Chiang's good graces.

Why did Chiang decide to raid this factory? There were several explanations at the time. One claimed that Chiang could tolerate opium but would draw the line at morphine and heroin. A second opinion ventured that Dai Li, the head of Guomindang intelligence and a beneficiary of narcotic funds, wanted more direct control of the proceeds of the factory for himself. After this short rupture, Du was able to talk his way back into favor, and he branched into the heroin market as well (Shanghai Municipal Police, November 25, 1933, D 5645; and February 5, 1940, D 9319).

Du clearly was taking advantage of the opportunity presented by the decreasing supply of European opiates. He inherited Eliopoulos's mantle, stepping into the market vacated by European sellers. What Eliopoulos may not have foreseen was that in the 1930s some Chinese-made morphine and heroin would begin to penetrate into the American market. One exporter who worked this route was Paul Crawley.

Crawley began his career in the California motion picture industry. He first went to Shanghai as a film distributor but later moved into his own variety of the import-export business. Crawley brought pianos and slot machines into China and sent heroin back to his brother in Los Angeles and to a gang of accomplices in San Francisco. Influential friends helped him bring the drug out of China. H. O. Tong, for instance, was one of his Shanghai business associates. A good person for a smuggler to know, Tong worked in the Shanghai Customs Bureau and was a close friend of Chiang Kai-shek's brother-in-law T. V. Soong (Shanghai Municipal Police, November 12, 1931, D 3057).

The relationship between Du and Chiang Kai-shek was mutually beneficial. Chiang continued to make efforts to control opium. In 1935 his government began a six-year plan to eliminate opium use. Du was named to the Shanghai Municipal Opium Suppression Committee. When we consider the pressures Chiang faced in 1935—Communist insurrection, Japanese invasion, opposition from factions within his own party—the appointment seems less a cynical or corrupt calculation than a rational opportunity to increase his control over strong warring forces. If we apply this lesson to the Taliban, we may be able to speculate that they faced a similar situation. Putting questions of revenue aside, the opium producers whom the Taliban were trying to control most likely were factionalized political actors in their own right. This may be part of the meaning of the "cultural differences" to which Noorullah Zadran alluded.

JAPAN CAPTURES THE NARCOTIC MARKET

Although Du Yuesheng ventured into heroin and morphine manufacture, it was his Japanese competitors who became the major producers of opiates for China in the 1930s. From the first, Japanese smugglers had been involved in bringing European pharmaceuticals to China, as can be seen in the statistics. Between 1898 and 1907 Japan imported an annual average of 20,000 ounces of morphine, which represents the standard of morphine consumption for legitimate purposes in the country. Between 1915 and 1920 the average increased to 495,000 ounces of morphine, about twenty-five times the legitimate amount ("Memorandum from the Anti-Opium Association," August 10, 1920, Foreign Office 317/5307/211; "Foreign Office to Board of Trade, March 23, 1921, Foreign Office 371/6593/162). When European supplies dwindled in the 1930s, Japanese manufacturers picked up the slack.

Until 1895 Japan had little experience with opium. In that year, however, Japan acquired the colony of Taiwan, which had a rich heritage of opium use. Faced with the sudden need for a practical opium policy, Japanese decision makers established a government opium production bureau, issued licenses for existing smokers, and taxed sales, hoping to control and eventually to discourage the use of opium. The architect of this policy was Goto Shimpei, who in 1895 was the head of the National Board of Health (Ryu 1983, 3–35).

Goto was an unlikely person to become entangled in international narcotics. He was born to a poor samurai family in 1857 and grew up during the excitement of the overthrow of Japan's feudal order. He received a degree in Western medicine, and his articles on public health earned him official recognition and an invitation to help create a modern public health service. Like Sir Malcolm Delevigne and Pino Arlacchi, Goto was a man with a larger social vision. He called his program "biological colonial management" (Tsurumi 1965, v. 1, 872). It included narcotics control.

Through the establishment of the opium monopoly, Taiwan, which initially had been an expensive drain on the Japanese budget, became self-supporting. The policy of gradual withdrawal, along with its monopoly apparatus, became the model used by the Japanese colonial system as it extended through Asia. Goto rose to become a politician of the first rank in early twentieth-century Japan, serving as Minister of Foreign Affairs, Minister of Home Affairs, and Mayor of Tokyo. He was a man of standing and integrity who never thought of himself as encouraging the international opium trade. Yet the system he fashioned leaked at the seams, creating opportunities for traffickers.

As Japan's Asian empire grew, its commercial outposts in and around China also served as staging areas for traffickers. Taiwan became a center of smuggling into south China. Korea, occupied by Japan after 1905 and annexed after 1909, played a similar role in the north. The Japanese presence also penetrated China's sovereign territory, through concession areas and railways. North China became a jurisdictional patchwork in which smugglers could work with ease because, as Japanese subjects, they had special treaty rights that rendered them immune to Chinese law (Minami Manshu Tetsudo Kabushiki Kaisha, Kaisai Chosakai Dai Go Bu 1934).

Periodic scandals exposed this situation. One such drama involved Hoshi Hajime, founder and president of Hoshi Pharmaceuticals. Hoshi came to the narcotic business in 1914, when, through the recommendation of Goto, he received the monopoly license to produce morphine for the Taiwan colonial administration. By 1921 British authorities suspected that Hoshi's firm was supplying to sources other than the legitimate markets. The British consul in Taiwan estimated that 3500–4000 jin (4655–5320 lbs.) of morphine from the Hoshi Pharmaceutical Company reached south China annually (C. Eliot to Lord Curzon, February 26, 1921, PRO, FO371/6594/10-1). These suspicions appeared to have been well-founded when, after pressure was put on the Japanese government by the British consular service, a Japanese customs agent discovered Hoshi's opium on a ship headed for Vladivostok without proper papers. Further investigations produced enough evidence that Hoshi had to stand trial for misconduct and was acquitted only on appeal (Hoshi 1971; Hoshi 1926; "Memorandum, Opium Scandal," *Japan Chronicle*, May 17, 1925, Pro FO 371/12527/108–12; P. Butler to Sir John Tilley, October 16, 1926, PRO FO 371/11714; FO 371/9248/141–47).

White drugs and smoking opium moved between Taiwan and the China coast through the agency of Japanese who had contacts with manufacturers in Japan and dealers in China. One such man was Harry Yamazaki, a sea captain who had learned the smuggler's craft from a Portuguese opium dealer. Yamazaki bought drugs in Taiwan and elsewhere, then sold them in China. In the 1920s and 1930s his customers were Japanese *ronin*. These adventurers—part samurai, part gangster, part patriot—had gone to China with idealistic intentions of aiding the Chinese in the 1911 revolution. However, as the republic collapsed, many drifted into the service of Chinese warlords for whom opium and narcotics became a source of income (Nitanosa 1977, 95–98; "Note on the Operations of a Syndicate," Shanghai, January 1925, PRO FO 371/10969).

In the early 1920s narcotics came to Japan from European sources as well as from Hoshi's factory. As the decade came to a close, however, Japanese merchants took advantage of the increasing cost and decreasing availability of European drugs. Japanese alkaloid chemists, trained in Europe, returned to work in factories scattered in concessions on the Chinese mainland. These firms kept costs low, produced close to their market, undercut the prices of their European competitors, and developed a better quality of smoking heroin. The price of morphine plunged from £100–120 per kilo in 1926 to £70 per kilo in 1928 (Yamauchi 1956; Eliopoulos 1932).

One such chemist was Yamauchi Saburo, who worked in Qingdao, Shandong province, for several years before setting up his own company in Dairen, Manchuria. Producers like Yamauchi sold their product to wholesalers, who in turn distributed it through a system of retail merchants—Korean or Japanese adventurers whose restless lives and political activities in Asia made them familiar with men who could help to distribute the goods. At first there was much competition among the heroin makers; later, the stronger knocked the weaker out of the market. Those smugglers who survived the competition were the ones who bought protection from the Japanese army.

A 1932 bond issue of ¥30 million for industrial development was secured by a pledge of anticipated annual revenues of ¥5 million from the opium monopoly in the Japanese puppet-state of Manzhouguo (see map 12.2). At this time, Yamauchi tells us, heroin makers donated funds to the military, often receiving decorations in return (Yamauchi 1956).

In 1934 the government of Manzhouguo invited Nitanosa Otozo, a "patriotic agriculturalist of Osaka," to visit and tender some advice. Nitanosa was a peasant with connections to Goto Shimpei. He first became concerned with opium supply in 1895, at the time of the acquisition of Taiwan. He contacted Goto and, with his support, began the experimental planting of opium poppies on his land outside of Osaka. Through the 1910s and 1920s he used the facilities of the board of health to increase the alkaloid content of his opium plants, clearly a move in preparation for heroin manufacture.

Nitanosa went to Manzhouguo to help make that nation "self-sufficient in opium" and to end its dependence on imports from Persia. Under his guidance, as the Japanese expanded into north China, suitable fields were turned over to poppies. From 1935 to 1936 poppy cultivation increased by 28 percent. In 1937 it increased by another 17 percent. Long after Goto passed from the scene, his legacy remained visible in a colonial structure that aided drug trafficking. Even when there were officials in charge who disapproved of the traffic and wanted the opium monopoly to function as it had originally been intended to do, the potential for abuse was hard to control (Nitanosa 1977, 64, 92).

North China became a haven for heroin supplied by both Japanese and Chinese manufacturers. One reporter paints a vivid description of the "white face houses" where heroin could be purchased in Beijing in the 1930s. Low-class places, located in the eastern and western districts, they were open from sunrise to the middle of the night and supported a continual traffic of pale-faced men and women. Their windows were covered with tattered newspaper. Outside, two or three rickshaws might be parked, each stripped of its cushions and lanterns, which had been pawned to support habits. The better heroin dens could be found in the north of the city. The windows of these houses had glass panes covered with white paper shades. These establishments were run by Koreans, who at that time were Japanese subjects (Ah Nan 1937).

A typical operation involved three people. The manager sat at the counter and acted as both cashier and pawnbroker. At his side sat his wife who doled out heroin from a bag, using a long-handled brass spoon. She leveled off the powder with a spatula, then emptied the portion onto a square of waxed paper. "Pull or stab?" she asked, to find out if the customer intended to smoke the heroin or inject it. If the customer indicated smoking, a pack of matches and a cigarette came with the price. If injection was desired, the heroin was mixed with morphine, because the product from north China was quite pure. Patrons went into a back room to enjoy their purchase. In the darkened room they lounged on the heated *kong*. Here and there the flair of a match would

Map 12.2
Japanese Expansion

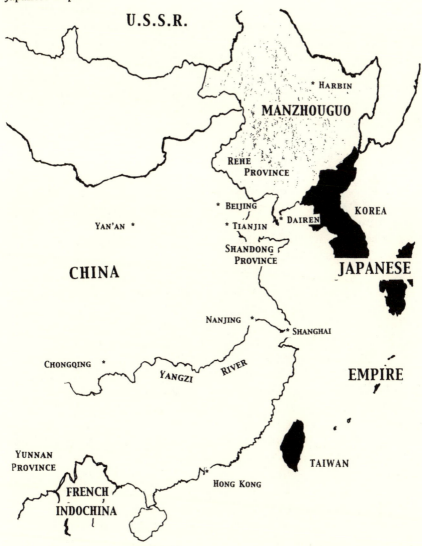

U.S.S.R.

* HARBIN

MANZHOUGUO

REHE
PROVINCE

* BEIJING

* TIANJIN

* DAIREN

KOREA

SHANDONG
PROVINCE

YAN'AN *

JAPANESE

CHINA

NANJING *

* SHANGHAI

CHONGQING *

EMPIRE

YANGZI   RIVER

YUNNAN
PROVINCE

TAIWAN

FRENCH
INDOCHINA

HONG KONG

outline a face in the gloomy room that stank of unwashed bodies and smoke (Ah Nan 1937).

THE FOG OF WAR

In the 1930s the delivery system for Chinese narcotics became professional, and heroin attracted more of the consumers that system served. Meanwhile, public attention was focused on the dramatic events that would lead the world into war. In North China reporters followed the Japanese army through a series of low-level conflicts as it expanded its control from Manzhouguo to the outskirts of Beijing (map 12.3). Just as today's news junkies are introduced briefly to names and places in the Middle East, only to find them eclipsed by pressing news stories closer to home, average Americans of the Depression years were diverted from following Asian events by their more immediate domestic worries. Once the North China situation escalated into war in 1937, earlier images were recalled, and when Japan became a U.S. enemy, its involvement in narcotics trafficking seemed appropriately sinister.

During World War II three responses made by the Japanese to their situation made that group of people seem then as cynical as the Taliban seemed half a century later. First, the Japanee armies marching south took over areas previously controlled by the Guomindang opium monopoly and Du Yuesheng's operation. Not only did those commanders need money, but they did not wish to cope with addicts in sudden withdrawal while they were attempting to control a hostile occupied population. As a solution, they reached for Goto's formula of opium monopoly. In 1939 the Japanese occupation authorities established the Ko-A-In, or Asia Development Board, to facilitate control of the Chinese economy. They attached an opium monopoly bureau to it. Commanders in charge of social control of occupied areas worried about continuing to supply their addicted population. In line with their general war supply problems, the Japanese faced chronic opium shortages for smoking and for opiate production. Manchurian supplies had been adequate to finance local growth during the period of low-level conflict in the north, because they had been buttressed by shipments from Persia. The war cut off that supplementary source of supply (Nakamura 1983).

Second, narcotics use in China was a reality that field commanders fighting a total war considered as part of their plans. I have found only one reference to the use of heroin as a way to weaken China, Yamauchi Saburo, a heroin maker who wrote his memoirs in the 1950s. Records from commanders at the front talk instead about undercutting Chinese sources of wealth: they used opium and morphine smuggling schemes to flood the market and drive down the price of Chinese opium. As the war progressed and inflation made currency all but useless, opium became a form of illegal tender that carried real value. It paid for both strategic materials and information impos-

Map 12.3
North China under Japanese Control

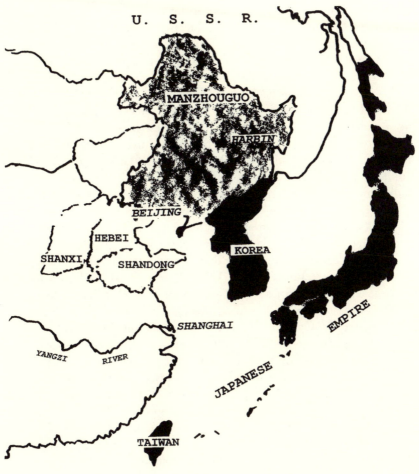

sible to acquire by using paper money (Yamauchi 1956; Yamamoto 1986; Okada 1980; Sunday *Mainichi*, December 9, 1984).

The Japanese were correct in assessing opium as strategic wealth. Once Shanghai fell to the Japanese, Du Yuesheng left for Hong Kong and, later, Chongqing, where Chiang Kai-shek and the Guomindang had retreated. While Du lived in semiretirement, part of his Green Gang operation worked against the Japanese under the direction of Chiang's chief of espionage, Dai Li, and his Military Statistics Bureau. Du and Dai created at least one company for the purpose of selling opium in Japanese-held territory to pay for much-needed supplies. Through this company, exchanges were facilitated by men like the shadowy Xu Caicheng, a double, or perhaps triple, agent whose name appears in police files and memoirs of the time as a Green Gang member, a Japanese espionage asset, a Chinese agent, and an opium merchant with a radio transmitter in his back room (Shen 1961; Zhang 1982).

A third condition the Japanese occupation forces faced was the appearance of anti-opium agitation among the Japanese residents of Manzhouguo. Confronted with official propaganda that touted the puppet state as a paradise where five races would live in harmony, many Japanese residents found it difficult to face the corpses of addicts that filled the streets of cities like Harbin and Mukden. In January 1937 a conference of Manchurian governors, who were Japanese, petitioned their government to reduce the number of opium shops and make it harder for addicts to get licenses. "The present conditions might be part of a plan to get rid of the weak," they said, but "it is a disgraceful reflection on the people that they should continue to take poison like candy" (Shen Ching Shi Bao, 1937, 59–60). This brought a belated effort by the local authorities to curb opium use through the local monopoly.

While the situation improved outwardly, much of the problem retreated to places like the Garden of Grand Contemplation. In spite of its poetic name, this garden was a jerry-built warren of flophouses located in the Chinese slums of Harbin, a city located in the northernmost region of Manchuria. The deserted building had been colonized by a thriving society that included displaced Chinese peasants down on their luck, heroin merchants, prostitutes, and a sprinkling of spies (Hinkosho Chiho Hoankyuko 1941).

The biographies of the residents of the Garden demonstrate the routes people followed into addiction and how heroin use blended in with opium use. Many tenants were peasants who had come north looking for work after floods and war had devastated their fields. Finding no employment, they turned to the slums and the solace available through a Japanese monopoly outlet located inside the Garden. Most addicts, however, found monopoly opium inferior, so they improved it by adding heroin, a practice called "silver inside gold." The heroin did not come from the monopoly, but it was in plentiful supply through resident smugglers, many of them Korean (Hinkosho Chiho Hoankyuko 1941).

Most of the Garden's residents could afford single rooms in one of the flophouses. Those whose habits brought them to the brink of death rented bunks in dormitories. Skin and bones, these unfortunates often had pawned even their clothes to support their habit. When they became sick and delirious, their fellow tenants tossed them into the bitter winter streets to freeze to death and stole what meager possessions remained. There were programs to help addicts. One resident took a cure, even though he was not an addict, to get the food and new suit of clothes that came with the process. Still, the scope of the problem facing the Japanese in 1941 in places like the Garden was beyond anything they could handle at the same time they fought a war (Hinkosho Chiho Hoankyuko 1941).

Satomi Hajime was a man with an excellent vantage point from which to make sense of the conflicts in Japanese drug policy. Satomi had gone to China in 1913 to study the language. He stayed, and became a journalist and a sales agent for the South Manchurian Railway. In 1937 he went to Shanghai, where he ran the city's opium monopoly for the Japanese army. At the end of the war he was designated a Class A war criminal and served time in Sugamo Prison. When questioned by American prosecutors, he gave them his perspective on the Japanese experience with narcotics. It was not entirely what they wanted to hear.

Satomi felt that the prosecutor wanted him to confirm that the Japanese command had been part of a larger conspiracy to traffic in narcotics. He could not do that, he said. Instead he told his interrogators that they should stop chasing after the big fish. It was the midlevel officials and officers who were involved in opium. When asked to comment on the Guomindang's supposedly successful campaign against opium in the 1930s, he replied that this assessment was mistaken and cited his own experience in Shanghai. When the Japanese army took over there, he said, they found a healthy opium market in spite of this campaign. He also contradicted the accusation that Japan was flooding China with opium from Manchuria. Satomi said that he had had to scramble for opium supplies because Manchuria could not meet the demand. The frustrated prosecutor asked if he realized that he had been violating international laws when he worked in Shanghai. Satomi replied, "Warfare itself is a violation of international law, and the violation of what I call the Opium Treaty was a necessary part of our warfare" (Satomi 1946).

Mr. Arlacchi should consider the words of Satomi Hajime. The good intentions of leaders can indeed be deeply held and sincere. At the same time, if the leaders also profess an ideology with larger political goals, short-term compromises might be made in order eventually to get those ideals into practice. Today's healthy heroin market continues to thrive on our political passions.

SUPPRESSION OF COUNTERREVOLUTIONARIES

When Pino Arlacchi went to Kandahar in 1997 to meet with the Taliban leadership, he discussed ways to improve their image in the world. He told them that two aspects of their image were in need of change: their opium trafficking and their treatment of women. Should the Taliban leaders indeed decide to undertake poppy eradication and narcotics reform, they could follow the precedent of the programs used by the Chinese Communist Party after its victory in 1949. The Afghani leadership could be influenced to seriously consider such a step by the argument that opium reform programs can be an excellent platform for the advancement of social revolution. Unfortunately, the part of their negative image that involves women is not so amenable to change because the social revolution that the Taliban envision is a regressive one, involving the regulation of ideas and the strict seclusion of women.

On October 1, 1949, the Chinese Communists emerged victorious from the Chinese revolution, and Chiang Kai-shek's Guomindang troops retreated to Taiwan. Like the other contenders in the struggle to control China, the Communist leadership had trafficked in opium during World War II. Desperate for funds, they had dabbled in the opium trade, though their philosophy decried drug consumption as a weapon of class and imperialist warfare. In February 1950 Zhou Enlai announced stringent opium control laws (Ch'en 1995; Ma 1993).

Satomi Hajime once said, "People who know China know no suppression campaign will work" (Satomi 1946). He had good reason to be cynical. Regulations had been promulgated before the Communist initiative, and no one was in a better position to appreciate how poor the results had been than Satomi. But the new Chinese regime was determined to make a clear distinction between themselves and the past. They looked hard for ways to make the laws work. While they had been holed up in the northern base camp during the war with the Nationalists, they had established a procedure for developing a dedicated Marxist corps of soldiers out of the ragtag volunteers who were drawn to their side. Based on the principle of "unity through criticism," the process involves self-criticism in a public forum. This activity has become familiar to us in the West through reports of the Cultural Revolution of the 1960s. In the early 1950s there was a mass movement called the Three Anti's/Five Anti's Campaign. Aimed at ridding China of the political corruption that had plagued the Nationalists, the Chinese Communist leadership included in this larger movement a national campaign against opium use (Ma 1993).

The program included the roundup, trials, and executions of notorious drug dealers. In addition, mass participation in anti-narcotics rallies, public confessions by ex-addicts, and neighborhood discussion groups molded popular opinion against drug use. During the time of this movement, China was at war with the United States in Korea. Drug peddlers could be identified with the Guomindang in Taiwan and, by extension, with the United States. This gave the movement a patriotic boost (Ma 1993).

The approach of the Chinese Communists in these campaigns appeared to be harsh but effective. They put forward the message that drug use was not only a degrading habit but also one that belonged to a decadent capitalist culture. The Taliban could use precisely this kind of propaganda program, substituting their brand of Islam for Chinese Marxism, but the Chinese campaigns, while successful in curbing drug use, also led to suppression of intellectuals and to larger human rights abuses. Considering the repressive social vision of the Taliban, such an anti-drug campaign would probably take the same direction. Is this a situation that international regulators would condone?

COLD WAR SOLUTIONS

The Chinese Communist leadership was successful in its anti-narcotics campaign because it could link opium and heroin elimination to a larger political program. In the early 1950s a war-weary Chinese population had been willing to give the new regime the benefit of the doubt, and so it could be inspired by a new vision. In the long run it became clear that the program of the 1950s had been successful only temporarily. Once Communist China reopened its markets to world trade, it rejoined the world's narcotic users as well. During the thirty years of its isolation, heroin had become the dominant opiate in the United States and Europe. At the end of the twentieth century China faced a growing heroin epidemic and found that its earlier approach to narcotics control was no longer so effective (Cheng 1993).

It is not surprising that today's heroin problem in China is centered in Yunnan. Not only does Yunnan have a rich legacy as an opium-producing territory, but just across its southern border lies the Golden Triangle, where the heroin trade continued to develop during the years of China's isolation. Because Mainland China was perceived as an enemy of the West, American propagandists found it convenient to blame China for the growing heroin traffic flowing into the United States from Burma and Thailand. Harry Anslinger, the longtime head of the Federal Bureau of Narcotics and a dedicated cold warrior, prominently accused the Communists throughout the 1950s of flooding the United States with heroin (Yates to Narasimhan, June 6, 1962, series 272, box 1, U.N. Archives, New York).

On May 31, 1962, Anslinger repeated this message as he addressed the seventeenth session of the U.N. Narcotics Commission in Geneva. This created a problem for members of the U.N. Opium Control Board. Gilbert Yates, the head of that body, privately worried about how to respond to the accusations. According to his information, it was Guomindang irregulars holed up in Burma, on the border with China, who were living off opium. Remnants of Chiang Kai-shek's armies driven out of China at the end of the revolution, in the early 1950s those soldiers had gone into the Burmese hills, where they staged several attempts to take back the Chinese mainland. After the failure of these efforts, they remained a force in local Burmese politics. It was here that the trafficker Khun Sa later developed his heroin empire (*New York Times*, June 1, 1962; Yates to Narasimhan, June 6, 1962; McCoy 1991, 162–78).

Yates was observing a shift from the old supply system that had been developed in China during the 1930s. After the Communist revolution in 1949 and the Guomindang retreat, most of the leadership of the defeated forces went to Taiwan, where they nurtured the rhetoric of reconquest of the mainland while building a new society on the island. Some, though, remained around the borders of China in a kind of unholy diaspora. One example is Ke Chaohuang. Ke had been a member of Dai Li's Military Statistics Bureau during the war. As such, he was assigned to infiltrate the secret societies in south China that had already been penetrated by the Japanese secret service. After the success of the revolution, he set up his own organization in Hong Kong, called 14K after the address of its headquarters. Soon 14K began trafficking in heroin from the Golden Triangle (He 1996).

This is the last lesson for Mr. Arlacchi. As the United States lobs missiles into Afghan territory, it is a good time to reflect on the conditions that have nurtured the narcotics trade network during the past century. The raw materials for narcotic production grow in places that not only are poor but also are strategically located near the conflicts that made that period so violent. Uneven economic development has been the foundation of much of the strife of the last hundred years, but alternative development requires political stability. How should development move forward? Who is to control the resources? Which traditional values and constraints must be sacrificed as the cost of modernization? Each of these questions is difficult to resolve in spite of our modern sophistication. Meanwhile, opium revenues have been too convenient a resource to be forsworn by those caught up in the wars and revolutions that modern tensions have spawned.

NOTE

1. Currency arrangements in China were complicated. In the 1930s China had a managed currency, the Chinese yuan, but foreign currency circulated in China as well. The symbol $ indicates Mexican silver dollars, which were popular and in which currency dollar values are given in this text. In 1930, U.S.$1.00 = Mex. $.3009 = yuan .2992 = £4.8621 = ¥.4939. U.S. Department of Commerce, *Statistical Abstract of the United States, 1932* (Washington: U.S. Government Printing Office, 1932).

REFERENCES

Adams, Walter. 1934. "Opium Situation in China." April 11. 893.114NARCOT-
ICS/708, U.S. State Department, RG 59, Box 7202, National Archives,
Washington, D.C.

Ah Nan. 1937. "White Face Houses of Beijing." In *Yapian Shi Jin Xi* [Opium today
and yesterday]. Edited by Tao Kangde. Shanghai: Yuzhoufeng She Chuban.

Ch'en, Jerome.1972. *Yuan Shih-k'ai*. Stanford, Calif.: Stanford University Press.

Ch'en Young-fa. 1995. "The Blooming Poppy Under the Red Sun: Yet Yenan Way
and the Opium Trade." In *New Perspectives on the Chinese Communist Revolution*. Edited by Tony Saich and Hans van de Ven. Armonk, N.Y.: M. E.
Sharpe.

Cheng Yi, ed. 1993. *Baise Youling: Zhongguo Dupin Newmu* [White ghost: The inside
story of Chinese narcotics]. Beijing: Guangming Ribao Chubanshe.

Courtwright, David. 1982. *Dark Paradise: Opiate Addiction in America Before 1940*.
Cambridge, Mass.: Harvard University Press.

Eliopoulos, Elie. 1932. 800.114N16 ELIOPOULOS/27, RG 59, Box 4536, National
Archives, Washington, D.C.

Financial Times, London.

Great Britain. Public Record Office, London, England.

Great Britain, Foreign Office. 1974. *The Opium Trade, 1910–1941*. Wilmington, Del.:
Scholarly Resources.

He Zengxiao. 1996. "Guangdong Hengmen Zhongyihui Shimo [History of the Hong
League]." *Zhonghua Wenshi Ziliao Wenku* [A treasury of Chinese source mate-
rials]. Beijing: Zhongguo Wenshi Chubanshe. Vol. 20, 366–83.

Hinkosho Chiho Hoankyuko [Hinko province regional police]. 1941. *Taikanen no
Kaibo* [Autopsy of the Garden of Grand Contemplation]. Kamminzoku Shakai
Jittai Chosatsu [Investigation into the social conditions of the Chinese race].
Mimeographed police report, labeled "Top Secret." National Diet Library,
Tokyo.

Hoshi Hajime. 1926. *Ahen Jiken* [The opium incident]. Tokyo: Hoshi Parmaceutical
Business School.

Hoshi Shinichi. 1971. *Jinmin wa Yowashi; Kanri wa Tsuyoshi* [The people are weak;
the bureaucrats are strong]. Tokyo: Kadokawa Shoten.

Hosie, Sir Alexander. 1914. *On the Trail of the Opium Poppy*. 4 vols. London: George
Philip.

Isaacs, Harold. 1951. *The Tragedy of the Chinese Revolution*. Stanford, Calif.: Stanford
University Press.

Ma Weigang. 1993. *Jinchang, Jindu: Jianguo Chuqi de Lishi Wenti* [Prohibit prostitution, prohibit poison: Historical problems from the early period of national
construction]. Beijing: Jingjuan Jiaoyu Chubanshe.

McCoy, Alfred W. 1991. *The Politics of Heroin: CIA Complicity in the Global Drug
Trade*. New York: Lawrence Hill.

Marshall, Jonathan. 1977. "Opium and the Politics of Gangsterism in Nationalist
China, 1927– 45." *Bulletin of Concerned Asian Scholars* 8: 19–48.

Martin, Brian. 1996. *The Shanghai Green Gang: Politics and Organized Crime, 1919–1937*. Berkeley: University of California Press.

Mei Zhen and Shao Pu (1987). *Haishang Wenren Du Yuesheng* [Shanghai celebrity Du Yuesheng]. Zengzhou: Henan Renmin Chubanshe.

Minami Manshu Tetsudo Kabushiki Kaisha, Kaisai Chosakai Dai Go Bu [Section Five, Economic Research Department, South Manchuria Railway Company]. 1934. *Manshukoku Ahen Seido oan* [Draft proposal for control of opium in Manzhouguo]. South Manchuria Railway Company archives, Library of Congress, Washington, D.C.

Minguo Ribao [Republican Daily]. 1916. July-August.

Moses, Sayas. 1933. 800.114N16 ELIOPOULOS/27, RG59, Box 4536, National Archives, Washington, D.C.

Musto, David. 1973. *The American Disease: Origins of Narcotic Control*. New Haven, Conn.: Yale University Press.

Nakamura Takahide. 1983. *Senji Nihon no Kahoku Keizei Shihai* [Japan's wartime economic management of North China]. Tokyo: Yamakawa Shupansha.

New York Times. November 25, 1997– July 17, 1998.

Nitanosa Nakaba. 1997. *Senso to Nihon Ahen Shi: Aheno Nitanosa Otozo no Shogai* [War and the history of Japanese opium: The life of Nitanosa Otozo, the opium king]. Tokyo: Subaru Shobo.

North China Herald. February 8, 1907–July and August 1916.

Okada Yoshimasa. 1980. "Chukoku Shihei Gizo Jiken no Zembo" [The complete picture of the Chinese currency counterfeiting caper]. *Rekishi to Jimbutsu* 110 (October).

Parassinen, Terry. 1983. *Secret Passions, Secret Remedies: Narcotic Drugs in British Society, 1820–1930*. Philadelphia: ISHI Press.

Riens, Thomas. 1991. "Reform, Nationalism, and Internationalism: The Opium Suppression Movement in China and the Anglo-American Influence, 1900–1908." *Modern Asian Studies* 25: 101–42.

Ryu Meishu. 1983. *Taiwan Tochi to Ahen Mondai* [Control of Taiwan and the opium problem]. Tokyo: Yamakawa Shoten.

Satomi Hajime. 1946. International Prosecutors Office, Interrrogation no. 59, Case 426 (March 5), International Military Tribunal. National Diet Library, Tokyo.

Shanghai Municipal Police (Criminal Investigation Division). 1916. IO 670. National Archives, Washington, D.C. October 29.

Sheng Ching Shi Bao. [Sheng Ching News] 1937. January 24. Document 9668, Exhibit 383. International Military Tribunal, National Diet Library, Tokyo.

Shen Zui. 1961. "Wo Suo Zhidaode Dai Li" [The Dai Li I knew]. In *Wenshi Ziliao Xuanzhuan* [Selected historical resources]. Vol. 22. Beijing: Zhonghua Shuchu.

Stilwell, Joseph. 1935. "Political Issues and Problems—The Narcotic Situation." 893.114NARCOTICS/1547, U.S. State Department, RG 59, Box 7202, National Archives, Washington, D.C.

Takasugi, Shingo. 1984. "Akuma no Boryaku" [The devil's strategy]. Series of articles. Sunday *Mainichi*. December 2–30.

Taylor, Arnold. 1973. *American Diplomacy and Narcotics Traffic, 1900–1939: A Study in International Humanitarian Reform*. Durham, N.C.: Duke University Press.

Times (London). 1920. March 27.

Tsurumi, Yusuke. 1965–67. *Goto Shinpei.* 4 vols. Tokyo: Keisoshobo. United Nations Archives. New York.

United States State Department. Record Group 59. National Archives, Washington, D.C.

Xiao Juetian. 1996. "Jiang Jieshi Jinyan de Neimu" [The inside story of Chiang Kai-shek's opium suppression]. In *Zhonghua Wenshi Zilaio Wenku* [Treasury of Chinese historical materials]. Beijing: Zhongguo Wenshi Chubanshe. Vol. 20, 650–58.

Yamamoto Tsuneo. 1986. *Ahen to Taiho: Rikugun Showa Tsusho no Nananen* [Opium and cannon: Nine years in the army's Showa Trading Company]. Tokyo: PMC.

Yamauchi Saburo. 1956. "Mayaku to Senso: Nitchu Senso no Himitsu Heiki [Narcotics and war: A secret weapon of the China war]. *Jimbutsu Orai* [Who's who]. October.

Yu Enyang. 1966 [1917]. *Yunnan Shouyi Yunghe Gunghe Shimo Ji* [Record of Yunnan righteous leadership in protecting the republic]. Reprint ed. Taipei: Wenhai Chubanshe.

Zhang Wuihan. 1982. "Dai Li yu Juntongpe" [Dai Li and the Military Statistics Bureau]. In *Zhijiang Wenshi Ziliao* [Historical sources for Zhijiang Province]. Zhijiang: Renmin Chubanshe. Pp. 104–07.

Zhang Zaichuan. 1986. "Xuanhu Yishi de Tang San" [The eminent Tang San (Tang Jiyu)]. In *Panlong Wenshi Ziliao* vol. 1, pp. 13–26. Yunnan: Kunming. Historical Materials Collection. Center for Chinese Studies Library, University of California, Berkeley.

Zhang Zheyong. 1985. *Shanghai Jindai Shi* [The history of modern Shanghai]. Shanghai.

13

Hip to Be High: Heroin and Popular Culture in the Twentieth Century

Jill Jonnes

Long viewed as our most feared and stigmatized drug, heroin also served, beginning after the end of World War II, as the rebel hipster's drug of choice. Using heroin showed the square world of wage slaves and upright citizens that you were one of the wild ones, part of an artistic avant-garde that scorned and actively transgressed the usual rules of conduct. Heroin users were not just part of an alternative subculture to mainstream America. Their embrace of illegal drugs meant they were actively oppositional, defying authorities by continually breaking the law. Of course, instead of living the hateful life of the wage slave, the transgressors might well end up living the beleaguered life of the heroin addict.

Shocking and defying authority, *épater la bourgeoisie*, pushing the envelope—Western pop culture has championed these as goals in and of themselves in recent decades, even as it has become ever more difficult to shock anyone in late twentieth-century America. It was striking in the 1990s to see how heroin—long the most "transgressive" drug—became defanged by pop culture to the extent that at times it was presented as just another "lifestyle" choice. By the mid-1990s, this transformation was so noticeable that the media had come up with the term "heroin chic." This article traces heroin's journey through postwar popular culture, examining how that transformation took place.

Heroin, introduced in 1898 by the Bayer Pharmaceutical Company as a powerful cough medicine, became a street drug used for pleasure sometime around 1910. By January 1914 a D.C. newspaper, the *Washington Defender*, published an article that described growing drug addiction nationally. An illustration shows a rather natty young man asking for heroin at a pharmacy. Later that year the federal Harrison Narcotic Act restricted heroin, which had been easily available, to use only through medical prescription. By 1916 the psychiatrist Pearce Bailey wrote in the *New Republic* that "the heroin habit is essentially a matter of city life. . . . The majority are boys and young men who . . . seem to want something that promises to make life gayer and more enjoyable. . . . It would almost seem that their desire for something to brighten life up is at the bottom of their trouble and heroin is but a means" (Bailey 1916, 315–16).

One of the few first-person accounts we have of this first heroin epidemic is that of fifteen-year-old Leroy Street (a pseudonym). The son of a postman, he was living in lower Manhattan when, in 1910, he first tried "happy dust," offered by a young man-about-town much admired by the neighborhood youth. Street came to typify the new-style heroin addict—city boys who gathered on stoops and in local pool rooms to use drugs socially.

When Street snorted his first "blow," he expected "something very stimulating, a feeling of excitement and joy. Instead, the reaction was much more insidious, a smug complacency that began to steal over me in the most delightful manner" (Street 1953, 13). After a month of using heroin, he was hooked—as were, eventually, about one hundred young men from his West Village neighborhood. Street used Bayer heroin tablets from small bottles: he crushed them and diluted them somewhat with lactose. Clearly there was something in the pharmacology of the drug, that feeling of "complacency," perhaps even superiority, that was very satisfying. The highly addicting nature of heroin, combined with the fact that there was no obvious or easy cure, soon made it a drug deeply feared by families and communities.

The new federal drug laws, however, combined with ever more stringent international agreements, so diminished the availability of heroin that American use and addiction declined steadily during the 1920s and 1930s. By the end of World War II, Washington viewed illegal drugs as a largely vanquished social problem. An aging cohort of opiate addicts were generally found in the criminal classes or the slums of northern cities.

Marijuana had not been included in the Harrison Narcotic Act. Starting in the 1920s, black northern jazz musicians developed a distinctive "hepster" culture that celebrated creativity, spontaneous pleasure, freedom, and excitement. They lived the fast life, with marijuana as their distinctive inebriant. Largely left out of the American Dream in racist America, the hepsters rejected the central tenet of Western civilization: "the subordinating and disciplining of present conduct in the interests of future rewards" (Finestone 1957, 7).

Before we go further, let us consider the etymology of the word "hip" used in the title of this article. According to David Maurer's 1936 study, "Argot of the Underworld Narcotic Addict," "hip" was drug slang that went back to opium smoking days, when those who spent much time lying about in opium dens became "hipped," meaning that they got calluses on their hips (Maurer 1936, 122). Consequently, someone who was "hip" was a drug user. The entertainer Cab Calloway would explain "hip" in his 1939 *Cat-logue* as meaning "wise, sophisticated, someone with boots on" (Calloway 1949). The "Boots on" phrase referred to southern blacks smart enough to abandon the cotton fields, put on shoes, and head north. So already the word "hip" was conflating two things: drug use and being wise.

The supreme hipster in 1950s America was the alto saxophonist Charlie Parker, a pivotal figure in this new subculture. A brilliant musician who helped invent bebop, he had picked up a heroin habit in the late 1930s at about the age of fifteen, when he was playing clubs in Kansas City, one of America's more wide-open towns. In New York City, Parker became known as a jazz genius, idolized for his virtuosity. "A lot of younger people were so amazed and fascinated by the likes of Charlie's playing," remembered a colleague, "that something told them inside that if they were to assume his personal habits that they could get close to him" (Chubby Jackson in Gitler 1985, 279). Parker never proselytized or encouraged heroin use. Nonetheless, heroin acquired a deadly cachet and glamour from association with his talent and persona. For the first time, heroin possessed a powerful, articulated cultural meaning, joining marijuana as an essential of the hip life. Hipsters used heroin, squares didn't. "Bird was a big junkie, and to be like Bird you had to be a junkie. I mean everybody smoked pot, but when it came to hard shit, it didn't really become popular, if that's the right word to use, until Bird and his emulators" (Frankie Socolow in Gitler 1985, 281).

Red Rodney was a jazz musician who played and toured with Parker. Much of his career was destroyed by heroin addiction. Heroin, he explained, "was our badge. It was the thing that made us different from the rest of the world. It was the thing that said, 'We know. You don't.' It [heroin] was the thing that gave us membership in a unique club and for this membership we gave up everything else in the world. Every ambition. Every desire. Everything. It ruined most of the people" (Rodney in Gitler 1985, 282).

Heroin as a hip drug now began to move out beyond the world of jazz, and onto the streets. This coincided with steadily rising heroin availability, as the French Connection gangsters gradually upped their loads. Claude Brown grew up in the Harlem of the 1950s, and his autobiography, *Manchild in the Promised Land*, describes heroin's rapid spread: "Heroin had just about taken over Harlem. It seemed to be a kind of a plague. Every time I went uptown, somebody else was hooked, somebody else was strung out . . . cats would say . . . 'Look here, I got some shit,' meaning heroin. 'Let's get high.' They would say it so casually, the way somebody in another community might say, 'C'mon, let's have a drink.' . . . I'd tell them, 'No, man, I don't dabble in stuff like that.' They'd look at me and smile, feeling somewhat superior, more hip than I was because they were into drugs" (Brown 1965, 187, 189). The black inner-city neighborhood soon would become the locus of the full-time heroin subculture.

The Beats were important vectors in moving heroin and drugs-as-lifestyle out of the black jazzmen hipster realm and into the white world. William Burroughs's drug of choice seems to have been morphine, but books like his *Junkie* and *Naked Lunch* gave more seriousness and cachet to hard-core drug use and addiction as attractive oppositional lifestyles. Burroughs, emulating the first drug memoir, *Confessions of an English Opium Eater*, revived the genre, which has regular new entrants. The transgressive life was now actively promoted as an attractive alternative to responsible adulthood.

Yet, because of the hard-to-ignore havoc heroin was creating in black urban neighborhoods and the highly publicized heroin deaths of 1960s and 1970s rock stars, when middle-class baby boomers flocked to drug use, they largely shunned heroin, viewing it as a highly dangerous, fearsome substance that could be used only with a needle.

But, starting in the late 1970s, we begin to see the emergence of a new heroin romance. In 1978, Jim Carroll published a memoir, *The Basketball Diaries*, which described his life in the mid-1960s as a young Manhattan teenager whose main activities were playing high school basketball; getting high, especially on heroin; and having sex. By the final part of the book, Carroll realizes he's addicted: "I got to do something to off that little voice, I can gladly take sore muscles but my mind can't handle that monkey back there. And I used to laugh at that corny monkey phrase, too, I had it under control" (Carroll 1978, 122). He speaks bitterly of some of his fellow addicts whose well-to-do parents send them to places away from drugs. "Then there's us street kids that start fucking around very young, thirteen or so, and think we can control ourselves and not get strung out. It rarely works. I'm proof. So after two or three years of control, I wind up in the last scene: strung out and nothing to do but spend all day chasing dope" (190). The book ends on this unpromising note, and yet we know Carroll prevailed somehow, because he is identified on the jacket of the book as the "renowned poet and rock performer."

Newsweek writer Karen Schoemer had this to say about the book: "I never tried heroin, but I used to think I wanted to. White, middle-class, just out of college in 1987, I read Jim Carroll's *The Basketball Diaries*, a cornerstone of modern heroin mythology: he made it seem like the ultimate rite of passage, a drug that made you funnier, wiser, cooler and full of hilarious stories about running wild on New York's Lower East Side." Schoemer asked an unidentified singer-songwriter off heroin six years, when he began using heroin. "Probably the day I put down *The Basketball Diaries*" (Schoemer 1996, 50).

Whether such books mean to or not, what they say to the larger culture is that cool people who become poets and rock performers use heroin. They pursue dangerous bohemian adventures, but ultimately that doesn't seem to hold them up. After all, look, they have wildly popular books. Of course, this doesn't begin to convey the reality of heroin for most people who become addicted, or the terrific struggle later to stay away from the drug.

In the 1970s, using heroin got yet another layer of meaning attached to it. Baltimore city councilman and Methodist pastor Norman A. Handy, Sr., first used heroin while serving in Vietnam in the late 1960s. He continued once back home in Washington, D.C. Handy rationalized his drug use as a revolutionary act, part of changing the world. But in the end, mainly he was in full-time pursuit of the drug. "I had lost everything, including my sanity. Half my teeth had rotted, my skin was pale gray and pock marks were all over my face" (Matthews 1998). Handy eventually found his salvation in religion.

This idea that using heroin was the ultimate act of transgression, a way to defy and rebel against square society, was well entrenched by the 1970s. Listen to the words of Manhattan photographer Nan Goldin: "Heroin was the social drug of choice in the seventies. I started shooting heroin when I was 18. I went out to find it. I wanted to be a junkie from about 15—it was an act of revolution, a way of being as unlike my middle-class upbringing as it was possible to be" (Jackson 1998).

Goldin photographed her crowd of Lower East Side friends, and her unsettling, tawdry images became highly admired in the New York art scene. By the time they were published as *The Ballad of Sexual Dependency* in 1986, many of those depicted had died of AIDS, contracted through needle sharing. Remember Nan Goldin, because she will prove to be important. This Lower East Side drug-art scene, with all its messages of heroin as hip, will start going mainstream.

The Story of Junk by Linda Yablonsky is billed as a novel, but it seems to be pretty much a memoir of her drug scene on the Lower East Side of New York in the go-go 1980s before the 1987 Wall Street crash. Parts of it are also extremely similar to Nan Goldin's life. The two women certainly know each other, since Goldin did the jacket photo for *The Story of Junk*.

In the book, Yablonsky talks about her central character's "heroin honeymoon": "[When a college friend asked], 'How do you stay so young looking?' 'Heroin,' was my answer. He was a newspaper reporter and was accustomed to asking questions. He wanted to know what the drug did for me. I told him it calmed my nerves, relaxed my features, and lifted my spirits—in other words, kept the aging process at bay. 'Wait a minute,' he said, 'Are you telling me heroin is the fountain of youth?' 'Well, yes,' I said. 'Heroin cures everything'" (Yablonsky 1997, 192).

Later, as her life spirals relentlessly down, the main character reconsiders, musing, "Heroin plays with your soul—or whatever makes a person uniquely appealing and distinguishable. Like an enveloping shadow dissolving day into night, it sneaks across your vision and tries to put it out, whatever that joy is by which you live, it creeps inside and pushes you down, making you smaller and smaller, a tiny flame burning down" (232).

Like *The Basketball Diaries*, *The Story of Junk* ends with the main character still deeply involved in drugs. There is no indication of what it took for these people to retrieve their lives sufficiently to produce their books. Are they, for instance, on methadone? If so, they don't say, because, of course, methadone use is not hip at all, but rather is an acknowledgment that opiates have proved stronger than you.

The advent of AIDS contracted through shared needles put a serious damper on the downtown Manhattan art world's romance with heroin in the 1980s. Nan Goldin explained, "The notion of self-destruction as glamorous became self-indulgent when people around us started dying: that romantic vision of the self-destructive artist, having to suffer or induce pain in order to work, that sense that creativity has to come out of euphoric crisis, or out of extreme excess, changed" (Goldin 1996, 145). But not for long.

Around 1991 the Colombians began trafficking in heroin, providing a drug of such high purity that you did not have to inject to get high. Moreover, the widespread, mistaken notion that if you only smoke or snort heroin, you will not get addicted meant many more were willing to try what was established in some circles as a fabled hip drug. Twice as much heroin as in the 1980s was flowing into the country, making heroin far more available. Heroin was back on track.

Meanwhile, out in the west in the early 1990s, there was a whole other heroin resurgence developing, coming out of the grunge band scene in Seattle. In 1990 Perry Farrell, lead singer of a band called (frankly enough) Jane's Addiction and a known heroin user, said, when asked about heroin, "I think it's great." Of course, the most high-profile grunge musician-heroin addict came to be Kurt Cobain of the band Nirvana. Cobain was known as a tortured soul who had had trouble coping with the huge success in 1991 of his band's *Nevermind* album. The next year, Cobain began using heroin. He committed suicide in 1994.

By the mid-1990s, music industry executives said they had never seen heroin use so rampant among bands. The number of top alternative bands linked to heroin through a member's overdose, arrest, admitted use, or recovery is huge. Jonathan Melvoin, keyboard player for Smashing Pumpkins,

ODed in New York in mid-1996. Other known casualties were Everclear, Blind Melon, Skinny Puppy, 7 Year Bitch, Red Hot Chili Peppers, Stone Temple Pilots, The Breeders, Alice in Chains, Sublime, Sex Pistols, Porno for Pyros, and Depeche Mode. Together, these bands have sold sixty million albums. There must be a great many kids aware of these musicians and their heroin use.

The hot-ticket movie of 1994 was Quentin Tarantino's *Pulp Fiction*. In the film's most lusciously photographed sequence, the hood played by John Travolta mainlines a hot shot of heroin and goes for a long, blissful drive. "Coke is dead as dead. Heroin is coming back in a big fucking way," Eric Stoltz as the dealer tells the John Travolta character. This was just the most noticed of a series of Hollywood drug films in the 1990s that included *Naked Lunch*, *Rush*, *Killing Zoe*, *Fresh*, and *The Basketball Diaries*.

In May 1995 *Playboy* ran an article titled "Heroin Chic," which introduced a new term, "heroin achievers": "They are hip, motivated, educated—and on dope." The article included quotes like this: "Most people I get high with have PhDs," the author boasts. "They're not street trash. They're more like corrupted intellectuals. Now there's a glamorous look to it. The glamorous people are doing it." Or a nightclub owner saying of heroin users, "Basically they're trying to experience in real life what film noir is about—that certain bliss that will inevitably lead to doom" (Ehrman 1995, 66).

In the summer of 1996, the superhyped British movie *Trainspotting* hit the screens. It was constantly likened to Richard Lester's movie *A Hard Day's Night*—allowing, of course, for a very different plot and theme and message. *Newsweek* had this to say: "It is a romance that is seductive yet repellent, terrifying yet hilarious, depressing and exhilarating. *Trainspotting* is a lousy piece of propaganda. But it is a masterful waltz on the wild side" (Leland 1996, 54).

Vogue quoted the film's director, Danny Boyle: "The big lie in most movies about drugs is that they make taking them seem like pure misery. But that isn't true or people wouldn't do it. People who take drugs usually enjoy it—it's a fucking good time. Welsh's book captures that. Even though the story gets much darker in the second half, we wanted the film to have the wit and vitality of the book" (Powers 1996, 58).

Jonathan Larson's musical *Rent* opened in January 1996 to rave reviews, an updated *La Boheme*, set on the Lower East Side in the 1990s, where the drug is heroin and the disease is AIDS. The liner notes to the recorded score describe several of the characters as junkies or ex-junkies. Critics noted that *Rent* was just *Hair* retrofitted for the 1990s. If that is so, it says something about how heroin and addicts, once forbidden and feared, are now just grist for a musical that has touring shows crisscrossing the country.

The idea of heroin as the ultimate hip and artistic drug was gathering force throughout the early 1990s. By the mid-1990s, it had spawned a fashion movement that was dubbed "heroin chic." You may recall the photographs of Nan Goldin, who documented her drug-using circle of the late 1970s. These were so admired that they inspired endless imitators. Fashion magazine editors reportedly asked specifically for "heroin pictures." *Playboy* quoted a Gaultier model: "Oh, heroin? It's beauty secret number one. Everyone in Paris and Milan smokes it," because it helped maintain the in-demand "waif" look.

In the fall of 1996 the Whitney Museum of Modern Art honored Nan Goldin with an exhibit called "I'll Be Your Mirror," which outlined the connections between her work and 1990s heroin-chic fashion photography. Goldin had become a leading fashion photographer, sought after by the *New York Times* and other major magazines for her particular brand of fashion photos. The *Times* fashion editor, Holly Brubach, whose pages featured their share of these zoned-out images, solemnly explained that the "new transgressive fashion photography" was about the way "beauty really looks." There were numerous defensive explanations about how this was all an improvement over traditional false, air-brushed images.

Nan Goldin, long since clean, explained, seemingly sincerely, that she did not wish to promote drug use by her pictures. She told one interviewer, "I want to tell them [kids] they can become androgynous and unconventional without heroin" (Laurence 1996, 26). *Newsweek* quoted one model who got hooked as saying, "They wanted models that looked like junkies. The more skinny and f—ed up you looked, the more everyone thought you're fabulous" (Schoemer 1996, 52).

Then, in May 1997, the *New York Times* ran a report, beginning on its front page, about the heroin overdose death three months earlier of the fashion photographer Davide Sorrenti. His mother, also a photographer, had been agitating since his death against heroin chic. Phoenix House director Mitch Rosenthal was quoted as saying about heroin chic: "They are communicating a message of acceptability. They are communicating that this is not dangerous: an informed or smart user who's got it together will know what to do. They are lowering the threshold for use" (Spindler 1997, B7).

A few days after this story was printed, at a White House drug policy meeting, President Clinton spoke out: "Many of our fashion leaders are admitting flat out that images projected in fashion photos in the last few years have made heroin addiction seem glamorous and sexy and cool. . . . Glorification of heroin is not creative, it's destructive, it's not beautiful, it is ugly. And this is not about art, it's about life and death" (Wren 1997, A-22).

One photographer reported that fashion editors were backing off. "They literally said, 'We're not looking for any heroin pictures. . . . They want everything positive and healthy" (Spindler 1997, B-7). In the meantime, heroin use was steadily rising, and first users were younger and younger. The "Summary of Findings" from the 1998 National Household Survey on Drug Abuse reported that for heroin, "the rate of initiation for youths from 1994 to 1997 was at the highest level since the early 1970s."

Which is not to say that popular culture stopped presenting heroin as the hip drug, the choice of the really cool and artistic. There was the 1998 film, *High Art*. Based on the reviews and stories about this film, it appeared to be yet another Nan Goldin spin-off. One of the leading characters was a formerly successful photographer on the Lower East Side who uses heroin. Meanwhile, Nan Goldin herself relapsed.

What, then, is one to make of all this? At present, we have a popular culture that is obsessed with celebrities and that still celebrates the transgressive. The more you push what's left of the tattered envelope, the more attention you receive. If you are an ambitious person seeking fame and attention, it probably helps to engage in bad behavior and make sure the press knows about it. And so you have artists and others retailing their drug experiences as daring rites of passage. However, most people are not artists, and there is the very real peril that for them heroin will turn out to be not a rite of passage but a way of life. We have not managed to disconnect heroin use from its role as a statement of transgression. Unfortunately, as we enter the new millennium, it still remains hip to be high.

REFERENCES

Bailey, Pearce. 1916. "Heroin Habit." *New Republic*, 6 (April 22): 314–16.

Brown, Claude. 1965. *Manchild in the Promised Land*. New York: Signet. Paperback ed.

Calloway, Cab. 1949. *Cab Calloway's Cat-logue*. Rev. ed.

Carroll, Jim. 1978. *The Basketball Diaries*. New York: Penguin.

Ehrman, Mark. 1995. "Heroin Chic: Drug's Resurging Popularity in Los Angeles, CA." *Playboy*, May.

Finestone, H. 1957. "Cats, Kicks, and Color." *Social Problems* 5 (July).

Gitler, Ira. 1985. *Swing to Bop: An Oral History of the Transition to Jazz in the 1940s*. New York: Oxford University Press.

Goldin, Nan. 1996. *The Ballad of Sexual Dependency*. New York: Aperture.

Jackson, Tina. 1998. "Elegant and Wasted." *Guardian*. May 25.

Laurence, Charles. 1996. "Through a Lens Darkly: Mother of 'Heroin Chic' Has Regrets." *Chicago Sun-Times*, "Show" section, October 13.

Leland, John. 1996. "Track Stars." *Newsweek*. July 15.

Matthews, R. G. 1998. "Norman Handy Sr. Helps Addicts from Experience." *Baltimore Sun*, August 3, p. A1.

Maurer, David W. 1936. "Argot of Underworld Narcotic Addicts." *American Speech* 11 (April).

Powers, John. 1996. "People Are Talking About Movies." *Vogue*, July.

Schoemer, Karen. 1996. "Rockers, Models, and the New Allure of Heroin." *Newsweek*, August 26.

Spindler, Amy. 1997. "A Death Tarnishes Fashion's 'Heroin Look.'" *New York Times*, May 20.

Street, Leroy, with David Loth. 1953. *I Was a Drug Addict*. New York: Arlington House.

Wren, Christopher S. 1997. "Clinton Calls Fashion Ads' 'Heroin Chic' Deplorable." *New York Times*, May 22.

Yablonsky, Linda. 1997. *The Story of Junk*. Boston: Back Bay.

Index

About the Editor
and Contributors

DAVID T. COURTWRIGHT, professor of history at the University of North Florida, writes about social, medical, and legal history. His books on the history of drugs include *Addicts Who Survived: An Oral History of Narcotic Use in America, 1923–1965* (1989), *Dark Paradise: A History of Opiate Addiction in America* (expanded edition, 2001), and *Forces of Habit: Drugs and the Making of the Modern World* (2001).

ROBERT L. DUPONT, M.D., is clinical professor of psychiatry at the Georgetown University School of Medicine and president of the Institute for Behavior and Health, a nonprofit organization. He was the first director of the National Institute on Drug Abuse (NIDA) and in 1973 became the second White House drug czar, as Director of the Special Action Office for Drug Abuse Prevention (SAODAP). His book *The Selfish Brain: Learning from Addiction* was published in 1997.

ANDREW GOLUB is a principal investigator at National Development and Research Institutes in New York City and the author of the textbook *Decision Analysis: An Integrated Approach* (1997). His research examines social problems in the context of developing effective and cost-efficient government policy and programs. For the past decade his particular research interests have been drug epidemics, drug use by adolescents, and the association of drug abuse with criminality.

JEROME H. JAFFE, M.D., a psychiatrist and pharmacologist in the Washington, D.C. area, has worked with problems of drug abuse for more than four decades as a clinician, teacher and researcher, and policymaker. Under the Nixon administration he was appointed as the first national drug czar, one of a series of government positions he has held. He has conducted research on opioid agonists and antagonists, barbiturates, cocaine, alcohol, nicotine, and drug abuse treatment and has published his findings in both academic and popular formats.

BRUCE D. JOHNSON is the director of the Institute for Special Population Research at National Development and Research Institutes, a nonprofit organization in New York City. During a thirty-year career in drug abuse research, he has conducted twelve major research projects for the National Institute on Drug Abuse (NIDA) and the National Institute of Justice (NIJ). His books include *Marijuana Users and Drug Subcultures* (1973) and *Taking Care of Business: The Economics of Crime by Heroin Abusers* (1985). He is one of the authors of the annual reports for the Drug Abuse Warning Network.

JILL JONNES, a historian and writer, lives and works in Baltimore. Her many publications include *We're Still Here: The Rise, Fall, and Resurrection of the South Bronx* (1986) and *Hep-cats, Narcs, and Pipe Dreams: A History of America's Romance with Illegal Drugs* (1996). She has served as consulting historian for the museum of the Drug Enforcement Administration (DEA) in Washington, D.C.

HERBERT D. KLEBER, M.D., is professor of psychiatry and director of the Division on Substance Abuse at the College of Physicians and Surgeons of Columbia University, and the New York State Psychiatric Institute. He received his medical training at Thomas Jefferson Medical School and served his psychiatric residency at Yale University School of Medicine. Dr. Kleber is the author or coauthor of more than two hundred papers, chapters, and books dealing with all aspects of substance abuse.

EGIL KROGH, JR., was deputy assistant to the President for foreign affairs in the Nixon White House. He also served as assistant director of the Domestic Council staff, executive director of the Cabinet Committee on International Narcotics Control, and White House liaison officer to the District of Columbia. He practices law in Seattle.

ROBERT MACCOUN is professor of public policy and law at the Boalt Hall School of Law, University of California at Berkeley. Earlier in his career, he was a behavioral scientist at the RAND Corporation. His publications in the area of drugs include work on illicit drug dealing, alternative drug laws, and harm reduction. He is co-author with Peter Reuter of *Drug War Heresies: Learning from Other Vices, Times, and Places* (2001).

KATHRYN MEYER teaches history at Wayne State University. Her primary research interests are crime in Asia and international narcotics trafficking. She is co-author with Terry M. Parssinen of *Webs of Smoke: Smugglers, Warlords, Spies, and the History of the International Drug Trade* (1998).

DANIEL PATRICK MOYNIHAN, four-term United States senator from New York, was ranking minority member of the Senate Committee on Finance, among other key congressional positions. A member of the Cabinet or sub-cabinet of four successive presidential administrations, he also served as a U.S. ambassador to India and U.S. representative to the United Nations. As co-chair of the Democratic Party Substance Abuse Working Group, he played a significant role in drafting and achieving passage of the omnibus Anti-Drug Abuse Act of 1988. He has spoken and written voluminously on the public health problem posed by drug abuse.

DAVID F. MUSTO, M.D., professor of psychiatry and of the history of medicine at Yale University School of Medicine, has been a pioneer in the field of the history of drug abuse and drug policy in America. He is author of *The American Disease: Origins of Narcotic Control* (1973), and his research interests include White House drug policy, alcohol abuse and prohibition, and societal responses to cocaine use.

PETER REUTER is professor in the School of Public Affairs and the Department of Criminology at the University of Maryland. For twelve years a senior economist at the RAND Corporation, he founded and directed the RAND Drug Policy Research Center. He is the author of *Disorganized Crime: The Economics of the Visible Hand* (1983) and, with Robert MacCoun, of *Drug War Heresies: Learning from Other Vices, Times, and Places* (2001).

SALLY SATEL, M.D., is a psychiatrist at the Oasis Drug Treatment Clinic in Washington, D.C., a lecturer at the Yale University School of Medicine, and a fellow at the American Enterprise Institute, specializing in health policy. She is the author of numerous articles in the scholarly and popular press and of the books *Drug Treatment: The Case for Coercion* (1999) and *PC, M.D.: How Political Correctness Is Corrupting Medicine* (2000).

RICHARD S. SCHOTTENFELD, M.D., is a professor of psychiatry at the Yale University School of Medicine and director of the Substance Abuse

Treatment Unit at Yale-New Haven Hospital. His research focuses on improving the availability and effectiveness of addiction treatment. Currently, he is investigating primary care– and physician's care–based treatments for heroin addiction.

WILLIAM L. WHITE, senior research consultant at the Lighthouse Institute of Chestnut Health Systems in Bloomington, Illinois, has worked in the field of addiction treatment for more than thirty years. He is the author of *Slaying the Dragon: The History of Addiction Treatment and Recovery in America* (1998), and his research interests include the evolution of addiction treatment and the evaluation of treatment approaches for special populations.